Register Now for Online Access to Your Book!

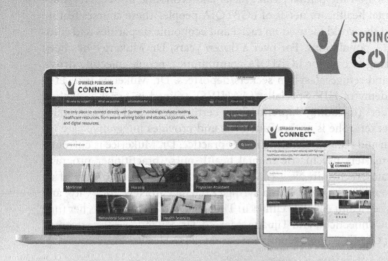
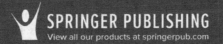

Ronica Mukerjee, DNP, MSN, FNP-BC, MsA, LAc, AAHIVS, teaches primary care at Yale University School of Nursing, having taught there since 2017. She is the program coordinator and creator of the Gender and Sexuality Health Justice concentration, focused on the primary care, racial and economic justice, HIV, substance use, and mental healthcare needs of LGBTQIA people. These courses feature experts from around the world focused on racial and economic disparities and clinical care in LGBTQIA populations. For over a dozen years, Dr. Mukerjee has been in practice specializing in care for LGBTQIA communities, people injecting drugs, HIV+ individuals, and refugees/asylum seekers/deportees. Dr. Mukerjee is a certified American Academy of HIV Specialist (AAHIVS), trained in facial aesthetics, substance use disorders (including Buprenorphine certification), and forensic evaluations for asylum seekers. She is an acupuncturist and provides integrative care incorporating Western and natural medicine in her practice. Dr. Mukerjee is currently enrolled in a post-masters psychiatric mental health nurse practitioner program. As owner of a private practice in New Haven, Connecticut; clinical director of an opioid overuse prevention program with a syringe exchange in New York City; and co-director of Refugee Health Alliance clinics in Tijuana, Dr. Mukerjee splits her time between New York, Connecticut, and Tijuana, Mexico. Dr. Mukerjee is the esteemed speaker for the 38th GLMA Annual Conference on LGBTQ Health.

Linda Wesp, PhD, MSN, FNP-C, RN, AAHIVS, is a clinical assistant professor at the University of Wisconsin Milwaukee College of Nursing and Zilber School of Public Health. She is an AANP board certified family nurse practitioner and certified HIV specialist through the American Academy of HIV Medicine. She has provided clinical care in community-based healthcare settings for LGBTQIA+ populations for over 16 years, with an expertise in transgender health and HIV. Dr. Wesp works nationally and internationally as an author, speaker, and educator about best practices and clinical guidelines in gender-affirming healthcare. Dr. Wesp is a member of the World Professional Association for Transgender Health Standards of Care Revision Working Group, as well as a Medical Advisory Board Member at the UCSF Center of Excellence for Transgender Health. Dr. Wesp obtained her bachelor of science in Nursing at Loyola University Chicago's Niehoff School of Nursing and her masters of science in Nursing at the University of Illinois Chicago College of Nursing. She completed her PhD in Nursing at the University of Wisconsin Milwaukee as a Jonas Nurse Leader Scholar, with a focus on participatory nursing research that improves access to healthcare and creates structural change to addresses health inequities among transgender and gender nonbinary youth of color. Dr. Wesp currently maintains a clinical practice focused on gender-affirming care and population health at Health Connections, Inc., in Milwaukee, Wisconsin.

Randi Singer, PhD, MSN, MEd, CNM, RN, is an assistant clinical professor at the University of Illinois Chicago College of Nursing. Dr. Singer obtained her bachelors degree at Clark University, her masters in Nursing from Vanderbilt University, and her PhD from Widener University. A CNM with a background in human sexuality, social justice, and equity education for healthcare providers, Dr. Singer's research and practice have focused on how reproductive and sexual health education through an equity lens can reduce health disparity for vulnerable and marginalized populations such as LGBTQIA+ pregnant and non-pregnant patients, sex workers, first generation Latinx adolescents, and pregnant teens. Although Dr. Singer has been teaching graduate nursing students at the University of Illinois at Chicago since 2018, she has been working in higher education since 2012 and has taught at Georgetown University, the University of Pennsylvania, and DePaul University Schools of Nursing. She has presented throughout the country on topics related to LGBTQ+ perinatal care and LGBTQ+ inclusive primary care. In collaboration with Sex Workers Outreach Project Chicago and Howard Brown Health, Randi Singer (PI) is currently funded by the Rita and Alex Hillman Foundation and the Institute for Research on Race and Public Policy at UIC to facilitate community empowered HIV/STI prevention interventions in Chicago, Illinois.

Dane Menkin, MSN, CRNP, is the divisional director of LGBTQ services at Main Line Health in Bryn Mawr, Pennsylvania, where he provides LGBTQ-specific clinical care with a focus on gender-affirming care for children, adolescents, and adults. Dane's role allows for access to a large healthcare system in the region to focus on an LGBTQ-competency curriculum implementation and workforce education. Dane is the recipient of the AANP Award for Excellence for PA in 2019. He is a member of WPATH and serves on the board of directors for The Jim Collins Foundation. Dane serves as adjunct faculty at Simmons University in the School of Nursing where he teaches graduate students advanced health assessment. He has presented across the country to healthcare and social service providers working with trans and non-binary clients and patients. Dane is a transmasculine-identified person and works hard to utilize that lens to inform both his practice and professional contributions.

CLINICIAN'S GUIDE TO LGBTQIA+ CARE

Cultural Safety and Social Justice in Primary, Sexual, and Reproductive Healthcare

Ronica Mukerjee, DNP, MSN, FNP-BC, MsA, LAc
Linda Wesp, PhD, MSN, FNP-C, RN
Randi Singer, PhD, MSN, MEd, CNM, RN

EDITORS

Dane Menkin, MSN, CRNP

CLINICAL CONTENT EDITOR

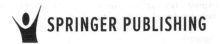

SPRINGER PUBLISHING

Springer Publishing Company, LLC
11 West 42nd Street
New York, NY 10036
www.springerpub.com
http://connect.springerpub.com

Acquisitions Editor: Elizabeth Nieginski
Compositor: S4Carlisle Publishing Services

ISBN: 978-0-8261-6915-0
ebook ISBN: 978-0-8261-6921-1
DOI: 10.1891/9780826169211

Supplemental materials are available at http://connect.springerpub.com/content/book/978-0-8261-6921-1.
Supplemental material ISBN: 978-0-8261-3928-3

21 22 23 24 25 / 5 4 3 2 1

The author and the publisher of this Work have made every effort to use sources believed to be reliable to provide information that is accurate and compatible with the standards generally accepted at the time of publication. Because medical science is continually advancing, our knowledge base continues to expand. Therefore, as new information becomes available, changes in procedures become necessary. We recommend that the reader always consult current research and specific institutional policies before performing any clinical procedure. The author and publisher shall not be liable for any special, consequential, or exemplary damages resulting, in whole or in part, from the readers' use of, or reliance on, the information contained in this book. The publisher has no responsibility for the persistence or accuracy of URLs for external or third-party Internet websites referred to in this publication and does not guarantee that any content on such websites is, or will remain, accurate or appropriate.

Library of Congress Cataloging-in-Publication Data
Names: Mukerjee, Ronica, editor. | Wesp, Linda, editor. | Singer, Randi,
   editor. | Menkin, Dane, editor.
Title: Clinician's guide to LGBTQIA+ care : cultural safety and social
   justice in primary, sexual and reproductive healthcare / editors, Ronica
   Mukerjee, Linda Wesp, Randi Singer; clinical content editor, Dane
   Menkin.
Other titles: Clinician's guide to LGBTQIA [plus] care
Description: New York : Springer Publishing Company, 2022. | Includes
   bibliographical references and index.
Identifiers: LCCN 2021000048 (print) | LCCN 2021000049 (ebook) | ISBN
   9780826169150 (cloth) | ISBN 9780826169211 (ebook)
Subjects: MESH: Sexual and Gender Minorities | Primary Health Care |
   Reproductive Health
Classification: LCC RA564.9.S49 (print) | LCC RA564.9.S49 (ebook) | NLM
   WA 300.1 | DDC 362.1086/6—dc23
LC record available at https://lccn.loc.gov/2021000048
LC ebook record available at https://lccn.loc.gov/2021000049

Contact sales@springerpub.com to receive discount rates on bulk purchases.

Linda Wesp: https://orcid.org/0000-0001-8520-6806
Randi Singer: https://orcid.org/0000-0001-9196-7812

Printed in the United States of America.

To Baby T.

Contents

PART III   SPECIFIC APPROACHES TO CARE

Contributors

Danielle Boudreau, CNM, WHNP-BC, is a sexual and reproductive nurse practitioner and nurse-midwife at Planned Parenthood of Northern New England. She works providing direct clinical care to people of all genders across the reproductive life span.

Sierra Bushe-Ribero, DNP, APN, CNM, WHNP-BC, is a clinical lead and certified nurse-midwife at the University of Chicago in Chicago, Illinois. She is a member of the Design Thinking Lab at the Center for Interdisciplinary Inquiry and Innovation in Sexual and Reproductive Health (Ci3), where she utilizes her expertise and experience to create curriculum and provide on-site support for healthcare providers that is inclusive of adolescents and LGBTQIA+ folks. She also provides full-scope midwifery care at University of Chicago Medicine and Saint Anthony Hospital in Chicago, Illinois. She has spent the past several years in the health realm providing sexual and reproductive healthcare to a variety of communities. She also is adjunct professor at DePaul University School of Nursing, where she teaches courses in Maternal Health, Culture, Ethics, Policy, and Health Promotion. Her practice research interest includes working to close healthcare disparity gaps in sexual, gender, and ethnic minority communities through the education of healthcare providers, staff, and students.

Jaymie Campbell Orphanidys, PhD, is a Black, queer, and transgender activist who has been working with and for Black and Brown lesbian, gay, bisexual, queer, transgender, and non-binary communities nationally for over 10 years. He is originally from Philadelphia but has a Bay Area vibe due to lifelong connections to California. Although Dr. Orphanidys is an introvert, he is not shy—he will eagerly skip small talk for deep conversations about anti-racism, intersectionality, Black Joy, the show *Grey's Anatomy*, and gender justice and liberation. Jaymie is a senior trainer for the Transgender Training Institute and Director of Training and Capacity Building at AccessMatters, a sexual and reproductive health nonprofit in Philadelphia, Pennsylvania. When Jaymie is not facilitating trainings, devising plans for dismantling white supremacy, or cultivating healing spaces for Black, Indigenous, and People of Color (BIPOC), he can be found heavily engrossed in a memoir.

Poonam Daryani, MPH, is a public health practitioner committed to health equity and social justice for historically marginalized communities. Her work focuses on the intersection of gender, sexuality, health justice, and human rights. Her background includes serving as a Clinical Teaching Fellow with the Yale Global Health Justice Partnership, reporting on the impacts of the 2015–16 Zika virus epidemic on caregivers in northeast Brazil, and teaching at a secondary school in Malaysia as a Fulbright grantee. Poonam holds a B.A. from Scripps College and an MPH from the Johns Hopkins Bloomberg School of Public Health.

Robin D'Aversa, MS, MEd, RN, is a DNP, CNM student at the University of Illinois at Chicago. They carry over a decade of experience in instructional leadership and teaching. They are committed to building highly resourced public learning institutions and communities in which civically engaged sexual and reproductive health curricula works to enlarge space for action and dialogue around equity. They labor for standardization of evidence-based sexual and gender minority (SGM)-affirming health curricula. They are dedicated to working with families, youth, and people in SGM communities toward educated and empowered choices in reproductive and sexual health.

Simon Adriane Ellis, MSN, CNM, ARNP, is a queer, trans, and non-binary identified certified nurse-midwife in full scope practice at Kaiser Permanente Washington in Seattle, Washington. Simon's clinical focus is on providing sexual and reproductive health services across the life span for people of all gender identities. They have clinical specialties in abortion care, LGBTQ family building, and gender-affirming care for transgender and non-binary people. Outside of the clinic, their advocacy work has included serving on the board of two reproductive justice organizations, co-authoring the Cedar River Clinics trans health toolkit, conducting original research on transgender pregnancy, and providing mentorship and training to students, clinic staff, and healthcare providers. Simon is also the gestational parent of their and their partner's super sweet kiddo, Irie Storm.

Julia Gelbort, MSN, RN, is a queer, non-binary emergency department RN working on Chicago's West Side. They entered the field of nursing with an undergraduate degree in Women's and Gender Studies and 10 years of experience as a sexuality educator and activist. Julia's nursing research and practice focuses on health equity in marginalized populations with an emphasis on harm reduction and community empowerment.

Ronni Getz, MSN, CNM, WHNP, is a Nurse-Midwife with Midwives @ Magee, University of Pittsburgh Medical Center in Pittsburgh, Pennsylvania. She earned a bachelor's degree in Gender and Sexuality Studies at Oberlin College. She earned her nursing and midwifery degrees from the Yale School of Nursing. She began her midwifery career as a Fellow with Midwives @ Magee and is now a full-time partner in the practice. Prior to becoming a midwife, she has worked in sex education, sexual violence prevention, and as a nurse at an independent abortion clinic. She is particularly interested in trauma-informed care and improving reproductive health disparities.

Kristin Keglovitz Baker, PA-C, AAHIVS, is the chief operating officer and certified physician assistant at Howard Brown Health in Chicago, Illinois. Her medical practice focus includes LGBTQ care, women's health, HIV medicine, health promotion, and interdisciplinary medical care for populations at risk. Kristin has been the driving force behind numerous projects at Howard Brown including alternative insemination, primary care opt-out HIV testing, rapid hepatitis C testing, and the expansion of service lines to include areas such as pediatrics, dental, and expanded sexual and reproductive health services. A physician assistant with a master's in Biochemistry, Kristin has been the primary investigator and subinvestigator on a number of clinical research trials, serves as Howard Brown's Institutional Review Board chair, and manages numerous grants as program director. Kristin is passionate about community health and improving health outcomes in communities of need.

Pia Pauline Lenon, BSN, RN, recently completed her nursing program at the University of Illinois at Chicago. Her nursing experience stems from a fast-paced progressive care unit, working with medical-surgical, cardiac, and intermediate patients. Her past research experience includes her senior capstone on breastmilk and low-birth weight infants and working as a research assistant on implementation-based science on HIV/STI research. More recently, she has worked as a research assistant regarding research on sexual and reproductive health and the LGBTQIA+ population. She is passionate about working to provide culturally safe care for marginalized populations.

Lazarus "Laz" Nance Letcher, MA, is pursuing a PhD in American Studies with a focus on folklore, Black liberation, and queer and trans studies at the University of New Mexico. They teach Introduction to Peace Studies, covering liberation movements and resistance efforts. They've written about topics like transgender and Two-Spirit migration, intersectional approaches to addiction and recovery, Black and Indigenous solidarity in liberation movements, and transgender connection/kinship through folklore. They give presentations like LGBTQ 101s with an emphasis on settler colonialism and white supremacy. They are the Health and Wellness Liaison at the LGBTQ Resource Center at the University of New Mexico. Laz is also a sexuality educator, wishing and working for a world where we all get what we desire.

D'hana Perry, MFA, BA, is the manager of TGNB Programming at Callen-Lorde Community Health Center in New York, New York, providing macro-level technical assistance and training to staff and outside agencies regarding transgender health access. They hold a BA in Sociology and Urban Studies from Ohio Wesleyan University and an MFA in Media Art from Emerson College. Perry has spent 20 years working in the nonprofit sector including time as an AmeriCorps volunteer, a legislative aide for a state representative, and a public health researcher at the Fenway Institute in Boston. Perry is also a professional DJ, video artist, and documentary filmmaker, whose work has been featured in various museums, galleries, and performance spaces. Perry is currently working towards an MS in Data Visualization at the Parsons School of Design.

Paige Ricca, DNP, MS, MBA, RN, is a Clinical Assistant Professor at the University of Illinois Chicago in Chicago, Illinois, and coordinates pediatric nursing and synthesis/leadership clinical practicums for undergraduate and graduate prelicensure students. She has over 20 years of experience of providing bedside care for infants, children, and their families in neonatal/pediatric intensive care, and pediatric emergency room settings. Her scholarly and education interests reflect her experiences as a nurse and a LGBTQIA community health advocate. She uses a population health approach to support students, faculty, and community members in their efforts to make spaces more affirming and inclusive for all, regardless of age, ethnicity, culture, religion, color, gender identity, sexual orientation, or physical or mental ability.

Liz Velek, MPH, has a master of public health from the Institute for the Advanced Study of Human Sexuality and a Sexual Health Education Certification from the University of Minnesota. She provides trainings and facilitates workshops on topics related to public health, sexuality, working with diverse sexual populations, and healthy sexuality. She is also a professional artist and a board member of Sex Workers Outreach Project, Chicago, Illinois.

Foreword

If you are a healthcare provider who seeks to practice social justice and patient-centered care while avoiding the "savior complex" trap, this book is your dream come true. As a queer AIDS activist, I entered the healthcare profession as an extension of my activism. I was fighting for and with my community for the right to knowledgeable, competent, respectful healthcare, so why not learn to provide that care myself? In 1993, less than a year after participating in an ACT UP die-in to pressure the local health system to open a dedicated healthcare center for people living with HIV, I entered PA school to learn the skills I needed to provide that care myself. While I received excellent training in clinical medicine, none of my classes focused on the social aspects of medicine, much less how healthcare could be a tool for justice. What I needed is exactly what this book provides: a framework and roadmap for providing care that is culturally safe and socially just.

As I write this text in the summer of 2020, the world is fighting another global pandemic that has no cure or vaccine. The U.S. government is attempting to rollback even the limited nondiscrimination protections that exist for LGBTQIA+ people in healthcare. And masses of people are mobilizing across the country to resist white supremacy, including a fierce cadre of Black trans leaders who refuse to bring anything less than their whole selves to the fight. I am grateful to the authors of this text for situating themselves unapologetically on the side of justice and providing a guide for each of us—LGBTQIA+ people, allies, and co-conspirators alike—to ensure that our clinical practice sees and supports the human rights of each person we encounter.

Tonia Poteat, PhD, MPH, PA-C, AAHIVS, DAAPA
Assistant Professor of Social Medicine
University of North Carolina at Chapel Hill

Preface

Dear Reader,

Thank you for picking up this book. We hope this guided exploration of gender and sexuality will provide you with a framework for providing clinical care that takes into consideration the social context we all live in—one where multiple historical processes of oppression continue to manifest as injustices in the healthcare setting and beyond. This text is intended to provide you with a perspective of providing clinical care for all people through the lens of racial, economic, and reproductive justice. Although not intended solely for clinicians, such as nurse practitioners and physician assistants, or public health workers practicing in the United States, this is the shared experience of the book's authors and editors. We provide examples, guidance, and case scenarios based on our collective experience as well as the most up to-date evidence-based guidelines for LGBTQIA+ (Lesbian, Gay, Bisexual, Trans, Queer, Intersex, Asexual, + more) patient populations; however, this text is not intended to be comprehensive on any topic related to LGBTQIA+ care. Rest assured, you do not need to read the book from cover to cover. You may decide to read only parts of certain chapters. We know, for example, that you may not be a clinician who does perinatal care, and you will not emerge as a perinatal care expert after referencing the perinatal chapter of the book. Instead, our hope is that you would emerge as a clinician who further understands both culturally safe contexts and care needed for LGBTQIA+ patients who are pregnant.

As most clinicians know, we are constantly navigating the ever-changing nature of evidence-based practice. By the time this text is published, some parts will already be outdated. Certain topics that are rapidly evolving based on emerging data, such as gender-affirming hormones or surgeries, were left intentionally broad and instead refer you to where you can find the most up-to-date guidelines. Thus, the book is not meant to be used as a stand-alone reference for medical care, but rather as a foundation for building an inclusive and justice-oriented practice. The book should be a tool that you use alongside a variety of other tools.

Language about gender, sexuality, intersex health, and asexuality will also always be in a constant state of necessary flux. Language must shift in order to frame ideas and change cultural concepts. Unfortunately, the culture of Western medicine and healthcare in the United States rarely attends to these cultural shifts closely enough, while also being decidedly oppressive at the roots. For example, federally funded research or electronic medical records will use terminology such as *Hispanic* or *Gender Identity Disorder* when for many community members, the correct terms may be *Latinx* or *trans*. Clinicians rarely learn about LGBTQIA+ history, systems of oppression, or racial/economic/disability justice in our foundational or continuing education. To begin to understand our LGBTQIA+ patients and care for them safely within the oppressive institutions that we work, we must pull from the humanities and social sciences, as well as community activism, to understand the realities of lived experience of our patients. This book introduces you to the multiple ongoing efforts to achieve health equity as well as racial, economic, and reproductive justice across multiple institutions, including healthcare. Our intention with this book is to provide you with a primer on some of these concepts, drawing from various resources that most clinicians are not aware of.

Why did you pick up this book? Perhaps because you are worried that the care you are providing lacks some fundamental pieces of knowledge. Perhaps you sense that you are not fully understanding your patients' lives or you want to expand your worldview, but you don't know where to start. Or perhaps you are passionate about social justice but didn't have time during nursing school to take all of the cool humanities classes. We, the authors and editors, encourage you to commit to your own transformation through learning. The more you understand the concepts woven throughout this book, the more you will catch up to your patients' lived realities and understand their clinical needs. As clinicians, we are often expected to never make mistakes. We encourage you to acknowledge that this will never be true. We must work to level the power dynamic during each patient encounter and the first step to doing this is recognizing that there is always room to learn and that our patients know more than we do about their lives and perspectives. It's also important for you to know that for the majority of patients there are rarely mistakes that you can make, beyond non-consensual transgressions, that are irreparable. Through careful self-examination and succinct heartfelt corrections and apologies, many patients can still feel heard and seen when you make mistakes. This is where we all must start.

We have so much work to do to improve the care settings for LGBTQIA+ patients and achieve health equity. Clinicians who wish to transform practice settings into LGBTQIA+-inclusive spaces are more likely to be successful if they use a community change process and collaborate with LGBTQIA+ advocates from a broad systems level perspective. We need more data, resources, and changes to public policy that address sexual and gender minority health. Eliminating health disparities among LGBTQIA+ populations and disrupting institutional oppression must start with you—the front-line clinicians. We hope this book can help you take some of these first steps and provide you with the resources you need to embark upon this work.

Also, if you read through this text and you think to yourself, *this book is missing a lot and needs revision and clarification,* you are not wrong. We aim to publish further editions that make this work more relevant, more human-rights focused, more culturally safe, more patient-centered, and more action-oriented in solidarity with health justice movements. We have every intention of caring for this book as much as we care for the health of our LGBTQIA+ patients. Many of the authors and editors identify as one or more of the letters in our acronym LGBTQIA+, while some are community allies—we are all dedicated to taking personal and collective steps toward achieving racial, economic, and reproductive justice.

We suggest an approach to care through various frameworks (see Part I: Frameworks) that are all primarily rooted in a cultural safety framework (Chapter 1). Cultural safety emphasizes patient-centered and community centered care that takes into consideration the intersecting and ongoing processes of oppression that impact LGBTQIA+ people every day—especially people of color. Clinical care, needs assessments, and resources must involve community members and provider-activists in order to identify which issues are important enough to warrant attention. Our work with patients and communities must incorporate appropriate and culturally safe language (Chapter 2), understand the roots and impact of stigma (Chapter 3), be anti-racist and eliminate microaggressions (Chapter 4), and be trauma-informed (Chapter 5).

Why did we choose the letter jumble of LGBTQIA+? This is an important question. Some activists/scholars/community members would only use LGBT or LGBTI, or even LGB and trans as separate. Some people would just say "Queer" and call it a day, or "Queer and Trans" to be as inclusive as possible. Well, we agree. Or maybe we disagree. It depends on your perspective. *Are labels useful or harmful?* This was a recurrent conversation that we maintained throughout this text. Couldn't we just write one giant chapter entitled *People Who Are the People They Say They Are* and another chapter called *People Who Are Into Other People in a Variety of Ways*? At the end of the day we chose to separate out the chapters in Part II into various chapters that comprise "People and Identities"—this was mostly because we couldn't figure out how to make it easily readable and navigable for clinicians searching for information regarding their patients. These chapters are rich in clinical scenarios and approaches to care that can be incorporated into your culturally safe practices.

The final part of the book dives deeper into several areas of clinical care that we hope you can apply to your practice immediately regardless of your area of expertise or specialization (Part III: Specific Approaches to Care). We have included a specific chapter on sexual healthcare (Chapter 10), which includes information about how to take a culturally safe sexual history, how to conduct a trauma-informed pelvic exam, information about supporting sexual function and pleasure for LGBTQIA+ people, and information about HIV and sexually transmitted infections. The final chapter focuses on perinatal care for LGBTQIA+ people (Chapter 11) and incorporates information about preconception counseling, prenatal visits, labor and birth practices, and postpartum care. This chapter also provides important information about pregnancy and postpartum care for transgender and gender expansive people, including information about chestfeeding that most clinicians have not otherwise had access to in our foundational training.

We sincerely hope that this book can expand your understanding of LGBTQIA+ populations and inspire you to be an accomplice in the fight for racial, economic, reproductive, and health justice. We need every single one of us to interrupt the processes of oppression and injustice that have fueled health inequities among various communities we discuss in this book. We hope these chapters provide you with some tools you were looking for, and perhaps some you didn't even know existed! Thank you for picking up this book and for creating a more culturally safe practice.

Ronica Mukerjee
Linda Wesp
Randi Singer

Acknowledgments

This book could not have been written without the work of Irihapeti Ramsden, who coined the term *cultural safety* and was seminal in defining it in Aotearoa (New Zealand). Her work sought to elucidate the inequity of power between healthcare professionals and the communities we serve. Without her work and the continuing work of Simon Brascoupé and the indigenous scholars who continue to push against the de facto imperialistic normalcy of healthcare systems around the world, we would not have a framework to envision the cultural safety of LGBTQIA+ lives. Although social justice is interwoven into cultural safety, we must also additionally acknowledge the work of so many queer and trans Black, Indigenous, people of color (BIPOC)-led movements throughout the world whose members have been excluded, separated, imprisoned, tortured, and murdered even as we/they work to change the culture of white heterosexual cisgender normalization that harms many types of communities. We, the editors of this book, write in the hopes of creating further momentum to increase the wellness and celebrate the lives of people whose lives are too often harmed or not properly bettered by their interactions with the healthcare systems that currently exist. In order for the health of all lives to properly matter, we must center the lives of people who have suffered the most from healthcare systems, including BIPOC LGBTQIA+ people. Thank you for helping us to continue to do that.

Frameworks

Cultural Safety Framework for LGBTQIA+ Communities

Ronica Mukerjee, Linda Wesp, and Randi Singer

LEARNING OBJECTIVES

By the end of this chapter, the reader will be able to:

- List three ways that cultural safety differs from cultural competence.
- Identify the five tenets of cultural safety that will be used throughout this book to frame care for LGBTQIA+ people.
- Self-reflect on personal biases that prevent provision of culturally safe care.
- List clinical care modifications supporting the cultural safety for LGBTQIA+ patients.

INTRODUCTION

Although many readers may be most familiar with the term *cultural sensitivity* or *cultural competence*, this text instead uses *cultural safety* to frame best practice recommendations. The idea of cultural sensitivity focuses on the basic awareness and willingness to learn about cultural differences.[1] The term *cultural competence* is perhaps what most clinicians are familiar with, and it is often used to describe provider awareness about the beliefs, values, and norms for various diverse groups of people and how we provide patient-centered care that respects differences in values, preferences, and needs.[2] These approaches, however, continually place the provider, not the patient, at the center. Culturally competent care was meant to be provided through a framework of patient empowerment.[3] Encouraging the examination of inherent power dynamics within the provider-patient relationship requires a strong theoretical foundation found to be lacking in cultural sensitivity and cultural competence frameworks.[4] Thus, these approaches are largely inadequate, especially for addressing the needs of marginalized groups, such as LGBTQIA+ communities.[4]

Cultural safety, however, reframes the cultural sensitivity and cultural competence approaches by building personal awareness and emphasizing patient-centered care. "Cultural safety involves understanding histories, safety needs, power imbalances and the influence of staff values and beliefs on service delivery."[5,6] Cultural safety is different from other frameworks because *safety* is defined by the patient rather than the healthcare provider. Cultural safety requires that healthcare providers prioritize the patient narrative, build community partnerships, and reflect upon the inherent existing power imbalances involved in patient care.[6] In order to achieve cultural safety, healthcare providers must seek out educational opportunities to guide personal, community and institutional growth while building strategic partnerships with LGBTQIA+ communities.[5,6] The authors of this text ask that you see beyond cultural sensitivity and competence and use the tools we provide to foster *cultural safety* for all patients (Figure 1.1).

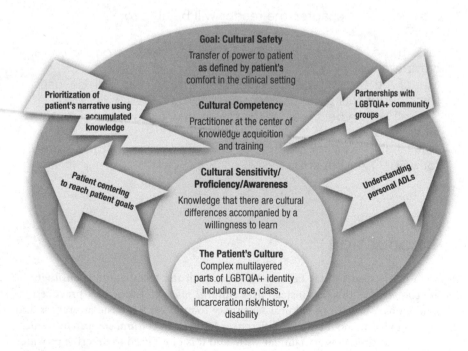

FIGURE 1.1 Connecting cultural competency to cultural safety. ADLs, activities of daily living.

OVERVIEW OF CULTURAL SAFETY

The goals of cultural safety go beyond recognizing disparities, and instead challenge systems that create inequality by focusing on provider-patient power dynamics as a source of this inequality.[7] To support the mission of this book, we have illustrated a model of cultural safety based on cultural safety literature. We describe cultural safety for LGBTQIA+ people using five main tenets that were adapted from the broader cultural safety literature.[4,7,8] These five tenets are: *partnerships, personal activities of daily living (ADLs), prevention of harm, patient centering,* and *purposeful self-reflection.*

More specifically, cultural safety seeks to form *partnerships* with patients in order to transfer power from the provider to the patient. It seeks to understand the patients' *personal ADLs* or everyday norms and experiences and incorporate them into clinical care. *Prevention of harm* is based on an understanding of what the patient needs to stay safe, with frequent check-ins from clinicians about whether the interactions or plan of care might inadvertently cause further harm. Also imperative for clinicians is to demonstrate *patient centering* by listening and providing meaningful care that fits into patients' lives. Finally, *purposeful self-reflection* is a process of uncovering one's own biases and beliefs that may lead to stigmatization or judgment, and transforming them so as to create a nonjudgmental environment.

Understanding clinical care through a cultural safety framework will provide a comprehensive approach to the management of the whole patient. This textbook will serve as a guide for clinicians in the management of LGBTQIA+ patients across primary care settings, sexual and reproductive health encounters, and urgent or emergency care. We will utilize a cultural safety framework to illustrate known barriers in accessing care for LGBTQIA+ patients. We will lean on this framework to demonstrate how the clinical needs of LGBTQIA+ patients are best met when care is approached through a cultural safety lens. What follows is a brief description of history of cultural safety, how it specifically applies to LGBTQIA+ patients, and an overview of the five major tenets of cultural safety used throughout this book.

ORIGINS OF CULTURAL SAFETY FRAMEWORK

Cultural safety was originally defined by Irihapeti Ramsden, a Maori Nursing Scholar working to ensure indigenous/aboriginal health equity.[8] Ramsden defined five major tenets of cultural safety as partnerships, protocols, process, positive purpose, and personal knowledge.[8] Overt, deliberate, and systemic change must be targeted and healthcare access and delivery must be improved for marginalized populations in order to create a space that is culturally safe for historically oppressed populations such as LGBTQIA+ individuals. Additionally, according to Ramsden, personal knowledge must include ongoing provider action shaped by self-reflection, and engagement or support of advocacy work that challenges and/or dismantles the provider's biases.[8] Finally, understanding historical and present day experiences of oppression is also a crucial component for enacting cultural safety.[8]

CULTURAL SAFETY AND LGBTQIA+ POPULATIONS

Based on these origins, it is important to examine closely the experiences of LG-BTQIA+ people in healthcare today. According to the Healthcare Equality Index (the national benchmarking tool for LGBTQ healthcare equality), LGBTQIA+ patients are, by and large, unhappy with the care they are receiving by their healthcare providers due to stigma and bias.[9] LGBTQIA+ patients avoid seeking healthcare services, or avoid full disclosure about their sexual orientation or gender identity rather than face the possibility of misunderstanding, discrimination, or even maltreatment by a healthcare provider. Of those surveyed for the Health Equality Index in 2014, 70% of transgender and gender-nonconforming respondents and almost 56% of lesbian, gay, or bisexual respondents had at least one of the following negative experiences[9]:

- Healthcare providers using harsh or abusive language
- Healthcare providers refusing to touch them or using excessive precautions
- Being blamed for their health status
- Healthcare providers being physically rough or abusive
- Patients being refused needed care

The clinical care that LGBTQIA+ patients want and deserve must not be prohibited by provider or institutional bias, cost of care, or lack of provider knowledge.[10-12] LGBTQIA+ patients deserve to receive healthcare that supports and decreases harm. End of story. Each tenet of culturally safe care, as described in the text that follows and illustrated in Figure 1.2, is essential.

Research suggests that many clinicians have little experience caring for LG-BTQIA+ populations.[13-15] This lack of experience impacts provider confidence to adequately care for patients identifying as LGBTQIA+, which leads to increased health disparities.[15] This book has been created as a guide to caring for LGBTQIA+ populations. To guide clinical practice, we use a cultural safety framework encouraging self-reflection and critical examination of interpersonal and societal power dynamics.[4] Care must reach beyond the low expectation of competency in order to best serve the needs of LGBTQIA+ patients.[4] "Cultural knowledge is important, but knowledge about how populations are marginalized is vital" (p. 97).[16] With that statement, Meleis and Im acknowledge that clinicians must be able to provide care informed by the narratives and history of oppression experienced by their patients.[16] Historical processes of oppression are fueled by ideologies that shape what is considered normal, and these processes subsequently create categories of individuals seen as "other," contributing to marginalization and inequalities.

THE DETRIMENT OF NORMALCY

Ideas of normalcy about sex, gender, and sexuality pervade healthcare and institutional spaces. Diagnoses produce categories of "health" versus "illness" that incorporate norms about gender and create systems of disciplinary power and reinforcement of racialized gender norms within our society.[17] In "Queer History, Mad History, and the Politics of Health" (2017), Kunzel[18] points out that medical systems have historically decreased autonomy and agency of LGBTQIA+ people by labeling common nonheterosexual, noncisgender identities as diagnoses or pathologies. Efforts to construct gayness as healthiness worked to align the definitions of modern lesbians and gays with gender normativity, supposed whiteness, and mainstream economic/relationship acceptability while showing all other types of queer/gay individuals as being the exception and representative of sickness and lack of health.[18] These ideas of normalcy and its associations with health continue to persist within healthcare. For example, LGBTQIA+ patients seen as "good" are contrasted with those who experience state violence, incarceration, institutional exclusion, racism, and other forms of prejudice. Kunzel clearly showcases how whiteness and economic stability in LGBTQIA+ populations is associated with "good" LGBTQIA+ identity while BIPOC (Black, Indigenous, people of color) populations are less likely to achieve that same status.[18]

Categories and ideas of normalcy create exclusion and lack of comfort for LGBTQIA+ patients including those with intersectional identities, such as African American trans women or same gender loving men of color or LGBTQIA+ people with disabilities as well as people who fall along the asexuality spectrum. Patients engaged in illegal activities such as sex work, despite the common cultural bias against such activities, will also face pathologization in healthcare settings due to ideas of normalcy.[18,19] As Spade and Willse state, "[b]y reconceptualizing how power works and attending to different forms of power, we can account for the seeming contradictions of systems where control occurs in multiple intersecting ways, including through processes of norm creation and enforcement that help us all see, experience and reproduce ourselves and the world according to racialized gender hierarchies" (p. 5).[17]

FIVE TENETS OF CULTURAL SAFETY FOR LGBTQIA+ POPULATIONS

With this understanding of the cultural safety framework and historical processes that contribute to lack of safety for LGBTQIA+ populations, what follows is an introduction to the main tenets of cultural safety we will use throughout this book. We will also discuss how culturally safe healthcare for the LGBTQIA+ patient will support health equity. Throughout the textbook, we will weave together details about how reproductive, racial, disability, and economic justice are impacted within these populations. We begin with outlining the five tenets of cultural safety, illustrated in Figure 1.2.

Tenet 1: Partnerships

Partnering with the patient and community provides collaborative care, and respects and incorporates patient knowledge and experiences as vital. When partnering with

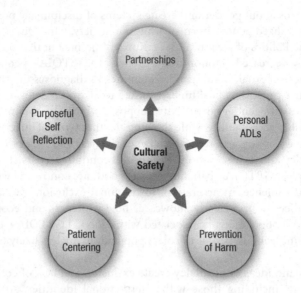

FIGURE 1.2 Cultural safety model for working with LGBTQIA+ populations.
ADLs, activities of daily living.
Source: Data from Ball J. Cultural safety in practice with children, families and communities. *Early Childhood Development Intercultural Partnerships.* Accessed November 19, 2019. http://www.ecdip.org/culturalsafety; Brascoupé S, Waters, C. Cultural safety exploring the applicability of the concept of cultural safety to aboriginal health and community wellness. *Int J Indig Health.* 2009;5(2). doi:10.3138/ijih .v5i2.28981; Ramsden I. Cultural safety. *N Z Nurs J Kai Tiaki.* 1990;83(11):18–19.

patients to achieve cultural safety, providers should work to unite with patients and the community in order to provide collaborative care and transfer of power to patients, while respecting and incorporating patient knowledge and experiences. With LGBTQIA+ communities, this means providing care for patients as partners in their care. How does "Partnering" look?

Tenet 2: Personal Activities of Daily Living (ADLs)

Personal ADLs include an understanding about the daily activities of life and survival that LGBTQIA+ individuals engage in as they face marginalization, stigma, and discrimination within society. Providers must explore and understand these experiences and the daily tasks that help people to resist and survive these challenges. In order to provide culturally safe care, clinicians must avoid asking patients to explain themselves, their practices, and identities in a way that resonates as invasive, ignorantly curious, or unnecessary. Researching about the various daily struggles that LGBTQIA+ people face and respecting ADLs is crucial. Avoiding asking unneeded, not-overly-curious questions about these practices helps to create trust between providers and patients. When working with patients whose gender identities or sexual practices may be unfamiliar to clinicians, be aware that various personal ADLs may be important to understand and discuss in a nonjudgmental way. For example, a norm for many trans men is chest-binding either before or instead of double mastectomy. Chest-binding can cause chest pain, muscle atrophy, or other musculo-skeletal complications.[20] Clinicians who are working toward cultural safety would support patients to achieve their desired gender presentation through this personal ADL of chest-binding, despite the risk of clinical complications.

Tenet 3: Prevention of Harm

Prevention of harm is patient-driven engagement that works to support a patient's journeys toward health. Providers should engage in mutual learning with frequent check-ins to make sure the plan of care is safe and appropriate for the patient's lifestyle. This means, for example, supporting LGBTQIA+ patients who may be engaged in underground economy jobs such as sex work and helping to decrease harm in patients' lives by offering more routine STI testing, prophylaxis medication such as PrEP, or expedited treatment. Or, with regards to the previous example of trans men doing daily chest-binding, clinicians can recommend activities such as stretching or massage to decrease muscular atrophy and pain from this practice. In each case the focus should and must be the patient's priorities, even though clinicians recognize that there may be complications as a result of these goals.[21]

Tenet 4: Patient Centering

Patient centering is when the practitioner provides the means to achieve healthcare goals as decided by the patient, and then helps the patient move toward their goals. When providers have aligned purposes with patients, to provide the means to achieve the goals that patients want and/or need, this solidifies clinicians as part of patients' positive moves toward their goals. Completing prior authorizations with insurance companies is a simple way of helping trans and gender expansive patients access gender affirming care. Supporting patients without judgment when they are in difficult relationships also supports patient centering.

Tenet 5: Purposeful Self-Reflection

Purposeful self-reflection is when the provider becomes aware of their own cultural beliefs, including reflecting on their own blind spots and internal biases. This requires self-reflection and processes of accountability to deal responsibly with these internal processes, so they do not interfere with the provider-patient relationship. Providers should develop a practice of self-reflexivity to develop awareness of innate, tacit, and biased cultural beliefs in order to address them. In the context of the powered provider-patient relationships, the onus of understanding cultural biases falls on the provider rather than the patient. With LGBTQIA+ patients (as with most patients), it may not be appropriate to speak these biases out loud but instead to eradicate their impact within the patient experiences.

ONLINE TOOLS FOR SELF-REFLECTION

- **Break the Prejudice Habit:** https://breaktheprejudicehabit.com/
- **LGBT Health Education Implicit Bias Guide:** www.lgbthealtheducation .org/wp-content/uploads/2018/10/Implicit-Bias-Guide-2018_Final .pdf
- **Hidden Bias Test:** www.tolerance.org/professional-development/ test-yourself-for-hidden-bias

ENACTING CULTURAL SAFETY WITHIN SPECIFIC LGBTQIA+ PATIENT POPULATIONS

What follows is a description of barriers to culturally safe care experiences by various LGBTQIA+ population groups, followed by brief examples of how the five tenets of culturally safe practices can be applied to benefit the health and well-being of LGBTQIA+ patients. Although groups are labeled according to commonly used identity terminology, we caution against assuming all people who describe themselves using a certain label will have identical or even similar experiences. Experiences of healthcare are influenced by the many identities that patients hold as well as the entrenched biases that systems, institutions, and providers have. This includes the resources available based on insurance and clinical/hospital access. Cultural safety approaches and considerations will be summarized at the end of each chapter throughout this book, providing greater detail about specific aspects of care and patient scenarios.

Several examples of the root causes of various barriers to culturally safe care for LGBTQIA+ populations include:

- Lack of understanding about gender diversity and the resulting assumptions about gender identity in relation to assigned-at-birth sex impacts trans people's ability to receive culturally safe care in all healthcare settings.[22,23]
- Assumptions about heteronormative sexual orientation and identity prevent lesbian, bisexual, and gay patients from receiving care that acknowledges their relationship experiences.[14]
- Lack of knowledge regarding innate diversity of human physiological and endocrinological differences, beyond the incorrect assumption that sex is binary, impacts the care of intersex patients.[24]
- Misunderstanding of healthy sexuality as driven by dominant ideologies about physical desire, romance, and marriage impacts proper healthcare of asexual patients.[25]

The following are some specific barriers for various groups of people in the LGBTQIA+ umbrella.

For People Who Are Trans, Nonbinary, or Gender Diverse: The barriers that trans and nonbinary people face in clinical settings have still not been fully addressed, despite the abundance of available guidelines.[11,26] Within the healthcare setting, trans patients report denial of care and verbal harassment, as well as lack of provider knowledge regarding appropriate gender-affirming interventions as barriers to revealing trans-status.[27] These barriers to care demonstrate the lack of cultural safety, especially a lack of patient centering and purposeful self-reflection that has led to a devaluation of trans people's narratives, needs, and experiences.[28–30] In this textbook, cultural safety will guide all aspects of the care of trans patients, including preventive care, hormonal care, surgical care, nonbinary and gender nonconforming identities, and fertility options, as well as some aspects of psychosocial well-being.

For Lesbians, Same Gender Loving/Attracted Women, Women Who Have Sex With Women, and More: For lesbian-identified people and women who have sex with women, care is often complicated by a lack of provider knowledge about the health needs for people who have experiences outside of the dominant heterosexual culture's understanding about sexual identity and behavior.[31] Dominant ideologies assume penile-vaginal or insertive-receptive sex is the norm, and anything outside of that is often misunderstood. Health needs for women, including trans feminine people, who have sex with women or lesbian-identified people must also include racial, cultural, and economic differences that impact their patient process.[31] Care that incorporates personal ADLs for same gender loving/attracted women might include asking questions about what types of sex a person is having, if and how toys are used, and what body parts go where during sex. Understanding what kind of sex people are having is crucial to understand what types of sexual health screening is appropriate or unnecessary. For example, a lesbian-identified patient may be of trans experience themselves, or have, for example, trans feminine or trans masculine partners; this changes some aspects of these lesbian-identified patients' care because patients may have unique fertility or contraceptive needs. Additionally, trans masculine patients may have similar health needs to same gender loving/attracted women.

For Bisexual/Pansexual Patients: Bisexual- and pansexual-identified people experience increased disparities in LGBTQIA+ communities due to the stigmatization of being attracted to people of various genders. Often bisexual and pansexual people are labeled as "promiscuous" or incorrectly as nonmonogamous, simply because they acknowledge attractions to multiple different types of people. People who identify as bisexual may find themselves hiding their identities or having their identities erased within the LGBTQIA+ community, and therefore less likely to access resources than gay- or lesbian-identified patients. Lifetime intimate partner violence (IPV) is greatest for bisexual women (56.9%) versus lesbian women (40.4%), and still higher than in heterosexual women (32.3%).[32] Provider knowledge of their bisexual patients can incorporate purposeful self-reflection when we address our own personal bias around assumptions about sexuality, as well as research or ask about struggles bisexual or pansexual patients may have around their identities and relationship experiences, including asking questions in a way that is both trauma-informed and validating.

For Gay Men, Same Gender Loving/Attracted Men, Men Who Have Sex With Men, and More: Gay men and men who have sex with men (MSM) patient populations experience health disparities in healthcare settings due to a stigmatization of their identities and sexual behavior, which is historically rooted in centuries of governmental control and legislation that criminalized specific sexual practices. Providers today still have a significant lack of understanding related to personal ADLs of the various types of sex, such as penile-anal and penile-oral sex. Lack of purposeful self-reflection leads to discomfort during the visit when these practices are discussed, inadequate screening and prevention, as well as a lack of culturally appropriate resources to support their lives and protocols.[14,31] African American MSM or same gender loving/attracted men receive a significant amount of public health focus because they are currently at greater risk for HIV acquisition due to ongoing processes of systemic racism that perpetuate barriers to HIV prevention, testing, and access to HIV care.[33] As a result, some communities of African American MSM have an increased viral load, making HIV transmission more likely, perpetuating significant health inequities in this population.[34] Partnerships with same gender loving/attracted men of color could include partnering with community-based organizations to understand specific needs and knowledges about barriers to care. Personal knowledge must include self-reflexivity about implicit biases around racial and sexual orientation stereotypes.[32] Trans masculine patients may also be men who are same gender loving/attracted men. Therefore, trans masculine people may require specific reproductive and sexual healthcare that often goes unaddressed. Understanding personal ADLs of all patients will ensure that screenings and other preventive measures are not missed due to provider assumptions.

For Asexual Patients: Asexual patients' identities and behaviors are not often understood or discussed thoroughly enough with asexual individuals by clinicians, once again, due to a lack of provider personal knowledge and personal ADLs, including sexual activity and relationship formations. For example, the self-identification, attraction, and behavior characteristics of asexual people may overlap but are distinct. The highest numbers of asexual individuals are noted when patients are asked about self-identification (71.3%) and lack of sexual attraction (69.2%) versus behavior.[25,35] Similarly in the push for "healthy sexuality," clinicians may lose sight of the pathologization inherent in seeing people with no need for sexual contact as disordered if patients themselves are not experiencing it that way.[35,36] Proper partnering will respect and incorporate patient knowledge, and for people who have asexual identities this can occur when providers respect asexuality as a valid identity and maintain nonjudgmental communication when discussing patient experiences.

For Queer Patients: When an individual presents for care and describes their identity as "queer," negative connotations or a lack of knowledge regarding this terminology may result in shock or surprise from providers unfamiliar with this term. The word *queer* is considered by many as an all-encompassing term to describe an aspect of themselves that is non-normative in one or more ways, usually describing sexual orientation or relationship structure. Queer might also describe gender identity, although it may often be referred to specifically as "genderqueer." Patient centered care means that there is an explicit lack of assumption about what a person might need in the way of healthcare simply because of how they identify themselves. It is important to understand that self-descriptive labels about identity are primarily a tool for understanding how a patient describes themselves, not a diagnosis that mandates a certain protocol of care. Rather, the culturally safe approach presented in this book encourages the provider to make space for asking about how a person identifies, but more importantly asking nonjudgmentally about patient practices (personal ADLs) and creating a plan of care that is appropriate and individualized (patient centered). Queer can be an umbrella term used by people who hold nonheterosexual or noncisgender identities.

Intersex Patients: Too often intersex patients are burdened with cancer scares related to their genitalia or gonads, even though we know the risks are low; thus, intersex people are subjected to unnecessary medical examinations. These practices are devoid of partnership with patients.[37] The pathologization and misunderstanding (lack of clinician personal knowledge) of intersex individuals' lives is central to the oppression that intersex patients have experienced in clinical settings. This is partially a result of a lack of understanding of the clinical implications associated with intersex status.[24,37,38] Likely, some of the clinical oppression that intersex patients experience is linked with overly curious invasive provision of care paired with conscious or unconscious othering by clinical providers. Intersex individuals may or may not identify with the LGBTQA patients depending on life experiences, identity, and/or personal preference. However, the possible medical history of nonconsensual genital surgeries and hormones, as well as the lack of understanding of the physiology and psychosocial needs of these patients, means that intersex patients may be lacking in culturally safe and conscientious care.[24,37]

LEGISLATIVE BARRIERS TO LGBTQIA+ HEALTH

Gender and identity have often been the subject of legislation, much of it since 2016, aimed at decreasing the rights that LGBTQIA+ people have. These laws are constantly shifting but are often shaped by federal and state legislation. We include several legislative examples in the text that follows that have impacted trans patients, individuals in the sex trade and street economies, undocumented LGBTQIA+ people, and those seeking access to abortion.

Protections of Trans Patients

State-by-state legislation regarding trans exclusion and discrimination vary wildly. Approximately 46% of LGBTQIA+ people live in states with high gender identity tallies, which indicate protections and freedoms related to "Non-Discrimination, LGBT Youth, Health and Safety, Ability to Correct the Name and Gender Marker on Identity Documents, and Adoption and Parenting."[39] The states with the most trans-inclusive legislation and policies are largely in the northeast and west coast of the United States, along with such states/territories as Puerto Rico, Minnesota, Colorado, New Mexico, and Illinois. More than half of LGBTQIA+ people (55%) live in the states with more restrictive and hostile policies; in fact, 28% of all LGBTQIA+ people are living in states with the most restrictive gender policies, with over two-thirds of trans people living without identification that matches their gender identity, often out of necessity related to their ongoing healthcare. Additionally, as of July 2019, 26 states in the United States have state Medicaid policies that negatively impact the care of trans patients.[39] These policies increase the lack of access to health and well-being that patients face while the inclusive policies within states with more trans-inclusive policies do not guarantee access to trans-inclusive providers, clinics, and other healthcare environments.

Intersecting Identities—LGBTQIA+ and Consensual Sex Working

Sex work is often a viable albeit stigmatized employment option for LGBTQIA+ people who have been excluded from institutional environments and other workplaces, are transiently housed, have experienced incarceration, or are otherwise left with few viable options for sustainable work. Research shows that stigma and discrimination experienced by transgender individuals contributes to a lack of economic opportunities. Transgender adolescents and young adults, for example, who have been ostracized by friends and family may end up running away from home and are more likely to exchange sex to generate income for rent, drugs, medicine, hormones, and gender-related surgeries.[40] Those who exchange sex may regularly experience the social repercussions of such stigmatized work.[40]

In the United States, the structural environment has recently become more detrimental to sex worker health and safety. Current political currents run counter to internationally accepted evidence-based human rights-informed best practice public health recommendations for the full decriminalization of sex work.[41,42] In April 2018, the Allow States and Victims to Fight Online Sex Trafficking Act of 2017 (FOSTA) (H.R. 1865—115th Congress: Allow States and Victims to Fight Online Sex Trafficking Act of 2017, 2018) was signed into law, creating an exception to section 230 of the 1996 Communications Decency Act, holding websites criminally responsible for third parties who advertise for prostitution on their platforms. Also in April 2018, the Department of Justice seized and shut down Backpage, an affordable online advertising platform that allowed sex workers to advertise their businesses, screen clients, and work independently indoors.[43]

These events have limited sex workers' ability to advertise for themselves on the internet, thereby exacerbating their financial insecurity and pushing increasing numbers of sex workers into higher-risk work environments on the streets and under the control of exploitative third parties.[43] As websites respond to FOSTA without knowledge of how it will be enforced, health promotion and safety information resources for sex workers are also being affected, limiting access to essential information when sex workers need it most.[44] Social, economic, and policy changes like these, which shift the dynamics of existing sex marketplaces, affect sex worker HIV/STI risk.[45]

The FOSTA/SESTA 2017 legislation ostensibly made it illegal to advertise sex trafficking, knowingly benefit financially from participation in a venture that advertises sex trafficking, and to engage in activities related to sex trafficking besides advertising, knowingly or in reckless disregard that sex trafficking is involved.[46] The legislation targets consensual sex workers more than it does traffickers. For example, in 2018 alone, trafficking increased in San Francisco by 170% while nontrafficked sex workers have been forced to work in more unsafe environments without the safety of internet traceability of customers.[47]

Immigration Policy

According to a 2013 Williams Institute report,[48] there are approximately 270,000 undocumented LGBTQIA+ people and about 640,000 immigrants with legal documentation in the United States; however, LGBTQIA+ people are often excluded in news coverage about immigration. The vast majority of undocumented migrants are Latinx, and among documented immigrants approximately one-third each of immigrants are Latinx and Asian or Pacific Islander. Additionally, approximately 10% of all DACA recipients identify as LGBTQIA+.[48] Beyond these estimates, very little is known about LGBTQIA+ people and immigration due to lack of safe and proper census data collection. When designating people as asylum seeking refugees versus immigrants who may or may not achieve legal citizenship in the United States, immigration decisions are minimal considering how lack of LGBTQIA+ safety in countries of origin may impact LGBTQIA+ people. Although immigration policy has often been exclusive at best, exclusion of LGBTQIA+ immigrants has been increasing in the last decade.[49]

Access to Safe Abortion

Many LGBTQIA+ people need access to safe abortion.[50] Often the same legislators fighting for LGBTQIA+ exclusions are the same legislators fighting against access to safe abortion. In this way, the battle for LGBTQIA+ rights echoes that of people choosing to access reproductive termination resources.

TACKLING BARRIERS

In order to tackle these barriers for LGBTQIA+ patients, clinicians must increase their own clinical personal knowledge, seeing LGBTQIA+ patients as partners in their own healthcare, and actively creating and engaging in policies that prevent access to conscientious care.[51] Addressing barriers to care for LGBTQIA+ patients may occur in clinical settings, with patients, with insurers, with institutional settings where patients may be working or receive services, as well as local governmental agencies. Additionally, providers' involvement in changing healthcare policy is crucial to increasing healthcare access for trans patients.

Intersectional identities should be seen as crucial to the health of the patient alongside evolving identities that may change or shift with patients' desires or needs.[4] For example, there are multiple scholars within LGBTQIA+ studies frameworks who explore sexual and gender variance experiences through a disability framework.[18,52]

Even beyond this, the intersectional identities within disability frameworks are not often well-understood or explored within clinical contexts. Conversely, much of the disability sexual orientation discourse is rooted in heterosexual identity.[52] As with the experiences of LGBTQIA+ people and those with disabilities, the experiences of LGBTQIA+ people with disabilities are poorly understood by healthcare providers and, therefore, so is sexuality and relationship-building. Additionally, the type of disability matters greatly when assisting patients with disabilities with their identity-validation and health goals. A patient with a central spinal cord injury or a neurodivergent patient or a patient with an amputation will have very different needs and will experience their involvements in dating, sexuality, and relationships differently. Some people may have intersectional disabilities or adjacent identities, such as deaf people, who often do not identify as having a disability.[52,53] In order to support patients with disabilities, providers must fulfill a narrative exploration with patients in order to make sure that our healthcare interventions meet patients' goals and that their access to services is bettered by receiving clinical care. Although this textbook will not focus on LGBTQIA+ people with disabilities, please note the highlighted areas that focus on special considerations for being in solidarity with disability justice movements within clinical settings.

HOW DO WE KNOW IF WE ARE PROVIDING CULTURALLY SAFE CLINICAL CARE?

Initially, it may be easier to recognize lack of cultural safety rather than the presence of cultural safety. A lack of cultural safety exists when practices demean, devalue, or disempower LGBTQIA+ patients' identities. A common example is the leveraging of hormone prescriptions as a way to reward HIV+ trans patients for taking their HIV treatment medications, thereby devaluing the trans identity of the patient. Additionally, many clinicians working with asexual patients may create a goal of "having healthy sex" for their patients, even though this might not be the patient's goal. This can disempower the patient from choosing their own progress and goals.[7]

As a clinician, you can take specific action steps toward creating culturally safe healthcare encounters by focusing on the tenets of cultural safety and the examples provided throughout this book. Reducing health disparities for LGBTQIA+ patients will require a concerted effort on the part of clinicians; cultural safety is one proposed framework that may help clinicians better advocate for and support their LGBTQIA+ patients. The cultural safety framework recognizes that knowledge regarding the disadvantaged social status of oppressed populations is missing from most available clinical care guidelines or healthcare practice.[8] Cultural safety is defined as an outcome, wherein LGBTQIA+ individuals' historical and personal narratives are recognized and valued by clinicians. Cultural safety is an outcome for patients produced largely through the application of cultural competence in the clinical setting and the active work of providers to decrease barriers when outside of the patient-provider setting.[53]

Cultural safety does not end with the patient visit. Providers and staff must engage in creating avenues for increased access to safe and legal employment options for

LGBTQIA+ patients. To promote culturally safe care, clinicians must be leaders. We must educate current and future care providers, as well as public and private insurers, about the medical and economic needs of LGBTQIA+ patients. We have a responsibility to challenge biased insurance coverage that impacts patients' abilities to achieve appropriate testing, hormonal, or surgical needs while challenging queer- and transphobia within the healthcare systems.[50]

CONCLUSION

The cultural safety framework recognizes that the current health disparities of LGBTQIA+ people is a result of their systemic oppression and denial of equality within the healthcare system. The clinician is an active tool in decreasing the harm of ongoing stigma when working with LGBTQIA+ patients, via equalizing the power dynamic within the provider-patient relationship.[7] Clinicians working with the cultural safety framework can look to the five tenets outlined in this chapter: partnerships, personal ADLs, prevention of harm, patient centering, and purposeful self-reflection. Clinicians are tasked with understanding LGBTQIA+ patients' goals, cultural practices of achieving these goals, and patient choices related to said goals.

Because the authors of this text are using a framework of cultural safety to support best clinical practices for LGBTQIA+ patient care, each chapter ends with cultural safety summary points. These points intend to weave the chapter content together through the five cultural safety tenets. Keeping cultural safety at the forefront of clinical practice guides clinicians in culturally informed, conscious, and mindful care that acknowledges a patient's narrative and history of oppression. Maintaining a mindful clinical practice brings LGBTQIA+ patients one step closer to health equity and justice.

REFERENCES

1. Foronda CL. A concept analysis of cultural sensitivity. *J Transcult Nurs*. 2008;19(3): 207–212. doi:10.1177/1043659608317093
2. American Association of Colleges of Nursing. Cultural competency in nursing education. Accessed November 19, 2019. https://www.aacnnursing.org/Education-Resources/Tool-Kits/Cultural-Competency-in-Nursing-Education
3. Douglas MK, Rosenkoetter M, Pacquiao DF, et al. Guidelines for implementing culturally competent nursing care. *J Transcult Nurs*. 2014;25(2):109–121. doi:10.1177/1043659614520998
4. Wesp LM, Scheer V, Ruiz A, et al. An emancipatory approach to cultural competency: the application of critical race, postcolonial, and intersectionality theories. *Adv Nurs Sci*. 2018;41(4):316–326. doi:10.1097/ANS.0000000000000230
5. Crameri P, Barrett C, Latham J, et al. It is more than sex and clothes: culturally safe services for older lesbian, gay, bisexual, transgender and intersex people. *Australas J Ageing*. 2015;34:21–25. doi:10.1111/ajag.12270

6. McEldowney R, Connor MJ. Cultural safety as an ethic of care: a praxiological process. *J Transcult Nurs.* 2011;22(4):342–349. doi:10.1177/1043659611414139
7. Brascoupé S., Waters C. Cultural safety exploring the applicability of the concept of cultural safety to aboriginal health and community wellness. *Int Indig Health.* 2009;5(2). doi:10.3138/ijih.v5i2.28981
8. Papps E, Ramsden I. Cultural safety in nursing: the New Zealand experience. *Int J Qual Health Care.* 1996;8(5):491–497. doi:10.1093/intqhc/8.5.491
9. Human Rights Campaign. Healthcare Equality Index 2019. https://www.hrc.org/hei/
10. Singer R. LGBTQ training for obstetrical care providers in two urban settings: an examination of changes in knowledge, attitude and intended behavior. Published March 2016. https://search.proquest.com/openview/9951081849d694ffbbb8965e261dbe13/1?pq -origsite=gscholar&cbl=18750&diss=y
11. James S, Herman JL, Rankin S, et al. *The Report of the 2015 U.S. Transgender Survey.* National Center for Transgender Equality; 2015.
12. Vaccaro A, Koob RM. A critical and intersectional model of LGBTQ microaggressions: toward a more comprehensive understanding. *J Homosex.* 2019;66(10):1317–1344. doi:10 .1080/00918369.2018.1539583
13. Boroughs MS, Andres Bedoya C, O'Cleirigh C, et al. Toward defining, measuring, and evaluating LGBT cultural competence for psychologists. *Clin Psychol (New York).* 2015;22(2):151–171. doi:10.1111/cpsp.12098
14. American Medical Association. Understanding LGBTQ health issues. Published May2018. https://www.ama-assn.org/delivering-care/understanding-lgbtq-health-issues#Policy%20 on%20LGBTQ%20Health%20Issues
15. Beagan B, Fredericks E, Bryson M. Family physician perceptions of working with LGBTQ patients: physician training needs. *Can Med Educ J.* 2015;6(1):e14–e22. https://www.ncbi .nlm.nih.gov/pmc/articles/PMC4563618
16. Meleis AI, Im EO. Transcending marginalization in knowledge development. *Nurs Inq.* 1999;6(2):94–102. doi:10.1046/j.1440-1800.1999.00015.x
17. Spade D, Willse C. Norms and normalization. In: Disch L, Hawkesworth ME, eds. *The Oxford Handbook of Feminist Theory.* Oxford University Press; 2018. doi:10.1093 /oxfordhb/9780199328581.013.29
18. Kunzel R. Queer history, mad history, and the politics of health. *Am Q.* 2017;69(2): 315–319. doi:10.1353/aq.2017.0026
19. Baral SD, Friedman MR, Geibel S, et al. Male sex workers: practices, contexts, and vulnerabilities for HIV acquisition and transmission. *Lancet.* 2015;385(9964):260–273. doi:10.1016/S0140-6736(14)60801-1
20. Peitzmeier S, Gardner I, Weinand J, et al. Health impact of chest binding among transgender adults: a community-engaged, cross-sectional study. *Cult Health Sex.* 2017;19(1):64–75. doi:10.1080/13691058.2016.1191675
21. Benoit C, Maurice R, Abel G, et al. 'I dodged the stigma bullet': Canadian sex workers' situated responses to occupational stigma. *Cult Health Sex.* 2020;22(1):81–95. doi:10.108 0/13691058.2019.1576226
22. Reisner SL, Bradford J, Hopwood R, et al. Comprehensive transgender healthcare: the gender affirming clinical and public health model of fenway health. *J Urban Health.* 2015;92(3):584–592. doi:10.1007/s11524-015-9947-2
23. Kellett P, Fitton C. Supporting transvisibility and gender diversity in nursing practice and education: embracing cultural safety. *Nurs Inq.* 2017;24(1):e12146. doi:10.1111/nin.12146
24. Frader J, Alderson P, Asch A, et al. Health care professionals and intersex conditions. *Arch Pediatr Adolesc Med.* 2004;158(5):426. doi:10.1001/archpedi.158.5.426

25. Scherrer KS. Coming to an asexual identity: negotiating identity, negotiating desire. *Sexualities*. 2008;11(5):621–641. doi:10.1177/1363460708094269

26. Hembree WC, Cohen-Kettenis PT, Gooren L, et al. Endocrine treatment of gender-dysphoric/gender-incongruent persons: an Endocrine Society* clinical practice guideline. *J Clin Endocrinol Metab*. 2017;102(11):3869–3903. doi:10.1210/jc.2017-01658

27. Cicero EC, Reisner SL, Silva SG, et al. Health care experiences of transgender adults: an integrated mixed research literature review. *Adv Nurs Sci*. 2019;42(2):123–138. doi:10.1097/ANS.0000000000000256

28. Roberts TK, Fantz CR. Barriers to quality health care for the transgender population. *Clin Biochem*. 2014;47(10–11):983–987. doi:10.1016/j.clinbiochem.2014.02.009

29. Ayhan CHB, Bilgin H, Uluman OT, et al. A systematic review of the discrimination against sexual and gender minority in health care settings. *Int J Health Serv*. 2020;50(1):44–61. doi:10.1177/0020731419885093

30. Safer JD, Coleman E, Feldman J, et al. Barriers to health care for transgender individuals. *Curr Opin Endocrinol Diabetes Obes*. 2016;23(2):168–171. doi:10.1097/MED.0000000000000227

31. Centers for Disease Control and Prevention. A guide to taking a sexual history. 2018. https://www.cdc.gov/std/treatment/sexualhistory.pdf

32. Brown TNT, Herman JL. Intimate partner violence and sexual abuse among LGBT people. 2015:32. https://williamsinstitute.law.ucla.edu/publications/ipv-sex-abuse-lgbt-people

33. Institute of Medicine (U.S.), ed. *The Health of Lesbian, Gay, Bisexual, and Transgender People: Building a Foundation for Better Understanding*. National Academies Press; 2011.

34. Centers for Disease Control and Prevention. HIV and African American gay and bisexual men. Published March 19, 2019. https://www.cdc.gov/hiv/group/msm/bmsm.html

35. Van Houdenhove E, Gijs L, T'Sjoen G, et al. Asexuality: a multidimensional approach. *J Sex Res*. 2015;52(6):669–678. doi:10.1080/00224499.2014.898015

36. Gupta K. What does asexuality teach us about sexual disinterest? Recommendations for health professionals based on a qualitative study with asexually identified people. *J Sex Marital Ther*. 2017;43(1):1–14. doi:10.1080/0092623X.2015.1113593

37. Cools M, Robeva R, Hall J, et al. Caring for individuals with a difference of sex development (DSD): a Consensus Statement. *Nat Rev Endocrinol*. 2018;14(7):415–429. doi:10.1038/s41574-018-0010-8

38. Jenkins TM, Short SE. Negotiating intersex: a case for revising the theory of social diagnosis. *Soc Sci Med*. 2017;175:91–98. doi:10.1016/j.socscimed.2016.12.047

39. Movement Advancement Project. Mapping transgender equality in the United States. Accessed November 19, 2019. http://www.lgbtmap.org/mapping-trans-equality

40. Boyer CB, Greenberg L, Chutuape K, et al. Exchange of sex for drugs or money in adolescents and young adults: an examination of sociodemographic factors, HIV-related risk, and community context. *J Commun Health*. 2017;42(1):90–100. doi:10.1007/s10900-016-0234-2

41. Centers for Disease Control and Prevention. HIV risk among persons who exchange sex for money or nonmonetary items. 2016. https://www.cdc.gov/hiv/group/sexworkers.html

42. The Joint United Nations Programme on HIV/AIDS. On the fast-track to end AIDS. 2016. http://www.unaids.org/sites/default/files/media_asset/20151027_UNAIDS_PCB37_15_18_EN_rev1.pdf

43. Amnesty International. Amnesty International policy on state obligations to respect, protect, and fulfil the human rights of sex workers. Published May 26, 2016. https://www.amnesty.org/en/documents/pol30/4062/2016/en/

44. Witt E. After the closure of Backpage, increasingly vulnerable sex workers are demanding their rights. *The New Yorker*. June 8, 2018. Accessed November 22, 2019. https://www

.newyorker.com/news/dispatch/after-the-closure-of-backpage-increasingly-vulnerable
-sex-workers-are-demanding-their-rights

45. Tierney A. Sex workers say they're being pushed off social media platforms. *Vice*. Published April 2018. https://www.vice.com/en_us/article/3kjawb/sex-workers-say -theyre-being-pushed-off-social-media-platforms

46. Chamberlain L. FOSTA: a hostile law with human cost. *Fordham Law Rev.* 2019; 5(87):2171–2212. https://ir.lawnet.fordham.edu/cgi/viewcontent.cgi?article=5598&context =flr

47. Steimle S. New laws forced sex workers back on SF streets, caused 170% spike in human trafficking. *CBS SF BayArea*. February 3, 2019. Accessed November 19, 2019. https:// sanfrancisco.cbslocal.com/2019/02/03/new-laws-forced-sex-workers-back-on-sf-streets -caused-170-spike-in-human-trafficking/

48. Gates GJ. LGBT adult immigrants in the United States. *Williams Institute*. 2013:11. https:// williamsinstitute.law.ucla.edu/publications/lgbt-adult-immigrants-us

49. Gruberg S, Rooney C, McGovern A, et al. Serving LGBTQ immigrants and building welcoming communities. *Center for American Progress*. Accessed November 19, 2019. https://www.americanprogress.org/issues/lgbt/reports/2018/01/24/445308/serving -lgbtq-immigrants-building-welcoming-communities/

50. Riley J. State laws effectively banning abortion significantly harm LGBTQ people. *Metro Weekly*. Published May 17, 2019. https://www.metroweekly.com/2019/05/state-laws -effectively-banning-abortion-significantly-harm-lgbtq-people/

51. Yarhouse MA, Sides J, Page C. The complexities of multicultural competence with LGBT+ populations. In: Frisby CL, O'Donohue WT, eds. *Cultural Competence in Applied Psychology*. Springer International Publishing; 2018:575–602. doi:10.1007/978-3-319-78997-2_23

52. Kimball E, Vaccaro A, Tissi-Gassoway N, et al. Gender, sexuality, & (dis)ability: queer perspectives on the experiences of students with disabilities. *Disabil Stud Q*. 2018;38(2). doi:10.18061/dsq.v38i2.5937

53. Lane HL. Do deaf people have a disability? *Sign Lang Stud*. 2002;2(4):356–379. doi:10.1353/ sls.2002.0019

2

Language and Communication With LGBTQIA+ Communities

Randi Singer, Linda Wesp, Dane Menkin, Paige Ricca, Sierra Bushe-Ribero, and Kristin Keglovitz Baker

---

LEARNING OBJECTIVES

By the end of this chapter, the reader will be able to:

- Understand the concept of implicit bias and reflect upon how that may affect one's own biases and assumptions related to care.
- Explain differences between concepts of sex, gender, gender expression, gender identity, and sexual orientation and the associated terminology.
- Utilize communication skills that are inclusive and welcoming to LGBTQIA+ populations.
- Understand how to utilize the terminology glossary throughout the reading of this text.

INTRODUCTION

Language and communication are crucial for establishing culturally safe environments of care for LGBTQIA+ populations. Despite efforts to increase graduate student knowledge and understanding about cultural safety for LGBTQIA+ populations, many providers enter the clinical setting with little experience or information about culturally safe communication skills. Our healthcare system operates within a hetero-normative and cis-normative approach to care, meaning that our policies and processes operate as if all patients are heterosexual and cisgender.[1,2] LGBTQIA+ populations continue to face stigma within healthcare settings, and despite efforts to remain neutral and nonjudgmental, lack of awareness or explicit discrimination still exists.[3,4] Healthcare providers and the direct care staff who assist in providing care can play a significant role in improving LGBTQIA+ healthcare by learning about their own biases, becoming aware of the systemic barriers to care that LGBTQIA+ patients face, and learning communication skills that create patient-centered care that is inclusive and welcoming.

IMPLICIT BIAS

Implicit bias acknowledges the influence of unconscious sets of associations assigned to given social groups based on dominant ideologies. For example, when caring for LGBTQIA+ clients, implicit biases may often be noted by avoiding topics of conversation that are uncomfortable or unfamiliar for the provider, spending less time interacting with a patient, neglecting to ask certain questions, and other subtle patterns of behavior that affect the patient-provider bond.[5] Implicit bias has been reported to have a negative impact on outcomes in health such as increased rates of depression or anxiety.[6] Further, experiences during medical school have been shown to contribute to these avoidance behaviors.[7] Once an individual better understands their own implicit bias, however, they can be better prepared to address such biases and engage more respectfully and receptively with their patients. The time for learning LGBTQIA+—appropriate terms should occur prior to engaging with the patient and should not occur during the actual visit. Before you continue reading, jot down your answers to the following questions.

1. What are some practices that make *you* feel comfortable in healthcare settings when you are a patient?
2. Have *you* ever felt misunderstood or devalued by the staff or providers at a medical office?
3. What scares *you* the most about seeing a care provider?

It isn't just our LGBTQIA+ patients that feel vulnerable and anxious. Many patients feel vulnerable when going to the healthcare provider because they are exposing their bodies and their medical and physical history. It can be intimidating even for people whose bodies conform more or less to the expectations that our healthcare providers have. Just imagine for a moment how intimidating it might be for someone whose body does not conform to what society considers "the norm." As discussed in the previous chapter (Chapter 1), ideas of normalcy are everywhere within our society and our healthcare system, yet these can be harmful to people who have been categorized as "not normal" by society in multiple ways. The more we understand about our patients' experiences of marginalization due to societal ideologies about normalcy, the more we can address issues of trust and power imbalance within the provider-patient relationship.

Let's take a look at a specific patient scenario to examine further some potential assumptions and implicit biases that you may encounter as a healthcare provider (see Case Study 2.1).

Case Study 2.1

According to your schedule the next person is a 34-year-old individual who presents, for the first time, to your office for an "annual visit" and has a feminine first name with an "F" gender marker. You open the door to the exam room, assuming you will be doing a Pap smear and breast exam, and encounter a person who is masculine-appearing and introduces themselves to you as Trey.

STOP, think, and acknowledge. What are your first assumptions or thoughts when meeting this person? When you received your training as a healthcare provider, to what extent were you prepared for this visit and interaction? What would you do/say next? What are your immediate facial expressions/body language? What are the first words that come out of your mouth? We will work on methods to approach this visit throughout the remainder of this chapter. The first order of business for LGBTQIA+ inclusive care is knowing what words are affirming and respectful, and what those words mean.

TERMINOLOGY

As healthcare providers, it is pertinent to have familiarity with culturally safe terminology and communication skills. Sex and gender are two terms that are commonly utilized synonymously, yet they are different. *Sex* is a biological medical term referring to a certain combination of gonads, chromosomes, external gender organs, secondary sex characteristics, and hormonal balances. Because this term is historically divided into "male" and "female," this category does not recognize the existence of intersex bodies[8] or the realities of the diversity of human anatomy that does not fit neatly into two boxes. "Intersex is a general term used for a variety of conditions in which a person is born with reproductive or sexual anatomy that doesn't seem to fit the typical definition of female or male"[9] (discussed in greater detail in Chapter 9). *Gender* or gender role has a culturally influenced definition that insinuates dissimilarities and "standards" between men and women, in regards to how they live, work, behave, and perform.[10] Gender norms and expectations permeate all aspects of society, with expectations about masculinity and femininity influencing behavior, clothing, and hairstyle, among other things.

Gender identity refers to an internal personal identification with cultural definitions of masculinity/man/boy/male, femininity/woman/girl/female, as well as neither, both, or other gender(s). Cultural definitions vary greatly over time and are influenced by ethnicity, religion, and cultural norms. One's understanding of themselves in relation to societally defined standards of gender may or may not be congruent with the sex assigned at birth.[8,11] *Gender expression* is the external translation of an individual's gender identity. Gender expression describes external characteristics and behaviors that are socially defined as either masculine or feminine, such as dress, grooming, mannerisms, speech patterns, and social interactions. Social or cultural norms can vary widely and some characteristics that may be accepted as masculine, feminine, or neutral in one culture may not be assessed similarly in another.[12]

Several other terms are important when understanding human gender diversity. *Cisgender* refers to individuals whose gender identity and sex assigned at birth are congruent and persistent. This term was created to take the place of addressing cisgender persons as "non-transgender."[10] *Trans or transgender** are descriptors to describe people who have a gender identity that differs from that which would be expected based on assigned sex at birth.[8] Transgender is an umbrella term used broadly; however, many other terms may more accurately describe an individual's identity and experience.[13] For example, *genderqueer* is a term utilized to describe individuals whose gender "varies from the traditional norm" and/or refers to persons who were assigned female or male sex at birth, but their gender identity is not congruent with either male or female.[10] Some other terms to describe individuals who do not identify as exclusively male or female include *nonbinary, gender bender, gender fluid,* and *gender minority. Gender nonconforming* (also seen abbreviated as GNC) are individuals whose gender expression does not conform to typical societal expectations of their sex assigned at birth.[10] *Gender expansive* is a term more commonly used in reference to youth who may or may not identify as transgender, but wish to express themselves by expanding the boundaries that traditionally limit their identity.[14]

Now that you understand different gender variations, it is important to stop and note that everyone has a gender identity and a gender expression. All people also have a *sexual orientation*. So, what exactly is sexual orientation and how is it different than gender identity? Sexual orientation describes the nature of one's sexual, romantic, and emotional attraction and/or desire for romantic and/or sexual connections with other people.[8] Sexual orientation variations include *lesbian*, which is a term used to describe female-identified people attracted romantically, erotically, and/or emotionally to other female-identified people.[8] The predominant term in Western culture to describe men attracted to male-identified people is *gay*, a term to represent male identity who are attracted to males in a romantic, erotic, and/or emotional sense. Not all men who are sexually active with men identify as gay. Hence, when it comes to describing behavior as it differs from identity, men who have sex with men (MSM) or same gender loving (SGL) may be the more appropriate term to use.[15] The term

---

*For the purposes of clarity and simplicity, the terms *trans* and *transgender* will be used throughout this book to refer to trans, transgender, nonbinary, gender nonconforming, gender expansive, and genderqueer people as a set, unless otherwise indicated. Non-transgender people will be referred to as cisgender.

gay may also be used to refer to the LGBTQIA+ community as a whole, or as an individual identity label for anyone who does not identify as heterosexual.[8] An individual who is bisexual is a person who is emotionally, physically, and/or sexually attracted to males/men and females/women and, often, to all genders of people. This attraction does not have to be equally split between genders and there may be a preference for one gender over others.[8] Queer is a reclaimed word that historically has been a derogatory term, but which some LGBTQIA+ people now use from a place of power and self-identity. This term can blur the boundaries between categories of sexual orientation and gender and can include gay, lesbian, bisexual, transgender, and other identities.[8] Queer identities will be discussed in detail in Chapter 6. Additionally, the term *asexual* is an umbrella term that refers to individuals who do not experience sexual attraction, although many varied terms may be used. See Chapter 7 for further discussion about asexuality.

We have designed the Gender and Sexuality Seahorse (Figure 2.1) to help illustrate the plethora of ways that each person might describe and experience each of these components in themselves. We chose the image of a seahorse because they are an example from nature that challenges our fixed binary thinking about gender and sexuality. Like seahorses, we people are meant to exist beyond the confines of the binary. Human sexuality includes a myriad of physical, romantic and emotional attractions—unique as each individual is regarding other aspects of themselves. As illustrated in Figure 2.1, the Gender and Sexuality Seahorse, gender and sexuality may shift or they may never shift, and they are experienced and expressed in various ways. As clinicians, we do not need to clinically interrogate someone's gender or sexuality, which may shift in different environments and according to a person's needs. We must understand that these aspects of self may vary from our expected practice. Gender is always what the patient says it is and should not be assumed. Sexuality can be emotional and/or physical, could include various practices such as BDSM (see Chapters 6 and 10), and may shift throughout one's life. For example, an individual may be assigned female sex at birth, identifies as transgender, and expresses themselves in a masculine way. Additionally, they may be romantically and erotically attracted to those who are gender fluid and do not have a penis.

LGBTQIA+ ACRONYM

LGBTQ is a common acronym for the lesbian, gay, bisexual, transgender, queer community.[8] At times, LGBTQ is documented as LGBTQIA+ to ensure inclusivity and acknowledgment of the expansive diversity that exists. Remember that sex, gender, and sexuality are different, so within this acronym are sexual orientation variations (lesbian, gay, bisexual, queer, and asexual), gender identity variations (transgender), and physical characteristics (intersex). The "+" can include an additional representation of questioning (describing an individual who is unsure about their sexual orientation and/or gender identity), ally, pansexual, and/or two-spirit.

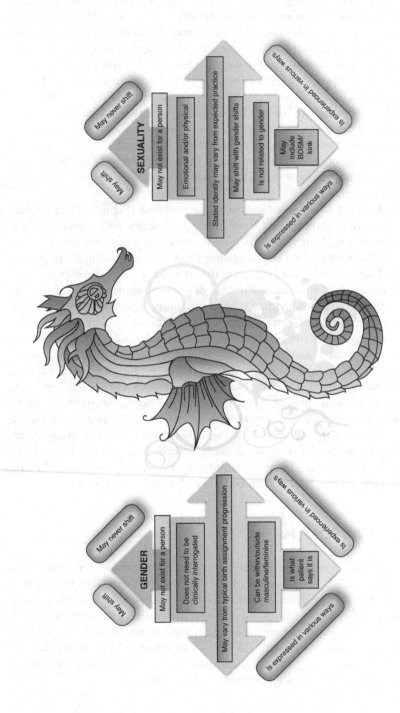

FIGURE 2.1 The Gender and Sexuality Seahorse.

Source: Courtesy of Ronica Mukerjee, 2020.

COMMUNICATION

First impressions are crucial for patients when establishing trust and safety in their clinician. Learning skills to provide patient-centered care and gaining awareness about structural barriers to care experienced by LGBTQIA+ patients is a step that healthcare providers can take toward health equity. As our world and the dynamic nature of language continues to evolve, it is reasonable to expect that the "+" will also evolve. The constant shifting levels of influence at social, political, or cultural levels, together with advances in sexuality and gender spectrum research, will play a role in healthcare provider individualized care and communication practices. Many times, a patient's plan of care also takes into consideration the family of origin and the chosen family. Therefore, it is essential to foster a holistic and trusting provider-patient relationship and environment by utilizing appropriate terminology with some familiarity, while remaining open to the inevitable evolution of language.

A crucial element of communication is to ask what gender-affirming terms patients use to describe themselves. Some individuals who are transgender may prefer the terms *transgender, trans, male, female, transman, transwoman, female-to-male* (FTM), *male-to-female* (MTF), *nonbinary, gender expansive, agender*, and a variety of other terms. Just as important as understanding how people describe themselves is asking for an individual's name and pronouns at the initial visit, and documenting this information so it is easily accessible. The initial introduction would be the ideal time to address the terms that are gender-appropriate for the specific individual, including how they feel most comfortable describing their body parts. All of this information can be noted in the electronic medical record. It is good practice to introduce yourself in the same way to every person you encounter, regardless of whether they express their gender in ways that might not be expected: "Hello, my name is Paige. I use she/her pronouns. Is there a name other than what's on your ID that you would like us to use for you while you are here?"

Case Study Revisited: Case Study 2.1

According to your schedule, the next person is a 34-year-old individual who presents, for the first time, to your office for an "annual visit" and has a feminine first name with an "F" gender marker. You open the door to the exam room, assuming you will be doing a Pap smear and breast exam, and encounter a person who is masculine-appearing and introduces themselves to you as Trey.

- How can you politely determine if you are in the correct room and what is needed for the "annual exam"?
- What is the best way to convey transgender patients' preferred names and pronouns used to all staff involved in their care, so it is clear how to communicate with the patient when providers or other staff walk into the room?

(continued)

Case Study Revisited: Case Study 2.1 (*continued*)

COMMUNICATION APPROACH:

Hey, nice to meet you. I use she/her pronouns, and you can call me Paige. What pronouns do you use? [Trey says, 'Sure, I use he/him.'] OK, great, Trey. What brings you in to see us today? It says "annual visit" in your chart but that can mean a lot of different things. What is most concerning for you to talk about today?

Prioritizing the patient's needs and concerns, and identifying name and pronouns, are important first steps in communication. If Trey says he is there for a Pap smear and breast exam, then further communication can happen to discuss and explain the procedures and what he might expect during the visit. Other considerations might include inquiries to the patient about whether the electronic medical record is correctly capturing the name and gender marker that is on the patient's insurance card. The provider or office staff can simply ask respectfully, "What name and gender marker is listed on your insurance card right now?" and explaining that this is important so that billing for the office visit and procedure can go smoothly. The provider or staff can explain that they will document the patient's name and pronouns in the record as well, but that billing information will often need to align with the name listed on the insurance. If the clinical setting has not set up policies and procedures around this, you can explain to the patient about steps being taken to ensure gender affirming care is provided throughout the clinical experience, including billing and lab services.

USING TERMINOLOGY GLOSSARY

The terminology glossary in the back of this book is structured to be used as you read through each chapter. When you come across terms with which you are unfamiliar, please flip to these pages and familiarize yourself with respectful and appropriate terminology. At the same time, remember to remain open to asking your patients how they describe and identify themselves because making assumptions about a patient based on a term defined in the glossary of a textbook does not support culturally safe practices. The only way to accurately describe an identity of an individual person is to ask them how they define themselves. These terms will always be more accurate than what you can find in this textbook or any other.

CONCLUSION

● Engage in purposeful self-reflection about your own implicit or explicit biases to enhance your ability to approach each person with a sense of open, compassionate, and respectful attitude. Doing this will transfer power to the patient as defined by their level of comfort in the clinical setting.

- Seek ongoing resources for expanding your understanding and knowledge of LGBTQIA+ populations, terminology, and cultures.
- Develop partnerships with LGBTQIA+ communities to enhance communication skills and understanding of language that is affirming.
- Practice patient centering through active and nonjudgmental communication, especially in clinical encounters where you are unfamiliar with the patient's life experience or identity.

REFERENCES

1. Grant MM. Learning, beliefs, and products: students' perspectives with project-based learning. *Interdiscip J Probl Based Learn.* 2011;5(2). doi:10.7771/1541-5015.1254
2. James S, Herman JL, Rankin S, et al. *The Report of the 2015 U.S. Transgender Survey.* National Center for Transgender Equality; 2015.
3. Baker K, Beagan B. Making assumptions, making space: an anthropological critique of cultural competency and its relevance to queer patients. *Med Anthropol Q.* 2014;28(4):578–598. doi:10.1111/maq.12129
4. Goins ES, Pye D. Check the box that best describes you: reflexively managing theory and praxis in LGBTQ health communication research. *Health Commun.* 2013;28(4):397–407. doi:10.1080/10410236.2012.690505
5. Phelan SM, Burgess DJ, Yeazel MW, et al. Impact of weight bias and stigma on quality of care and outcomes for patients with obesity. *Obes Rev.* 2015;16(4):319–326. doi:10.1111/obr.12266
6. Hall EV, Galinsky AD, Phillips KW. Gender profiling: a gendered race perspective on person-position fit. *Pers Soc Psychol Bull.* 2015;41(6):853–868. doi:10.1177/0146167215580779
7. van Ryn M, Hardeman R, Phelan SM, et al. Medical school experiences associated with change in implicit racial bias among 3547 students: a medical student CHANGES study report. *J Gen Intern Med.* 2015;30(12):1748–1756. doi:10.1007/s11606-015-3447-7
8. Green E, Peterson EN. *LGBTTSQI Terminology.* 2006. Accessed December 6, 2020. http://www.transacademics.org/lgbttsqiterminology.pdf
9. Intersex Society of North America. What is intersex? https://isna.org/faq/what_is_intersex/
10. Makadon HJ, Mayer KH, Potter J, et al, eds. *The Fenway Guide to Lesbian, Gay, Bisexual, and Transgender Health.* 2nd ed. American College of Physicians; 2015.
11. Dubin SN, Nolan IT, Streed CG Jr, et al. Transgender health care: improving medical students' and residents' training and awareness. *Adv Med Educ Pract.* 2018;(9):377–391. doi:10.2147/AMEP.S147183
12. Human Rights Campaign. Sexual orientation and gender identity definitions. 2015. http://www.hrc.org/resources/entry/sexual-orientation-and-gender-identity-terminology-and-definitions
13. Singer R. LGBTQ training for obstetrical care providers in two urban settings: an examination of changes in knowledge, attitude and intended behavior. Published March 2016. https://search.proquest.com/openview/9951081849d694ffbbb8965e261dbe13/1?pq-origsite=gscholar&cbl=18750&diss=y
14. Mountz S, Capous-Desyllas M, Pourciau E. "Because we're fighting to be ourselves:" voices from former foster youth who are transgender and gender expansive. *Child Welf.* 2018;96(1):103.
15. Gamarel KE, Brown L, Kahler CW, et al. Prevalence and correlates of substance use among youth living with HIV in clinical settings. *Drug Alcohol Depend.* 2016;169:11–18. doi:10.1016/j.drugalcdep.2016.10.002

3

Impact of Stigma

Danielle Boudreau, Robin D'Aversa, Julia Gelbort,
Ronica Mukerjee, Randi Singer, and Liz Velek

LEARNING OBJECTIVES

By the end of this chapter, the reader will be able to:

- Discuss the ways that LGBTQIA+ patients have experienced stigma throughout history.
- Describe the ways that incarceration affects the health of LGBTQIA+ Black, Indigenous, people of color (BIPOC).
- Understand the health disparities experienced by trans women of color.
- Discuss perinatal morbidity and mortality disparities for Black communities in the United States.
- Identify ways health can be negatively impacted by poverty.
- Define key ways Medicaid eligibility and exchange subsidies are allocated.
- Discuss differences between private and government insurance plans regarding coverage of transgender-related healthcare services.

INTRODUCTION

History shows us that stigma does not just happen; it is born out of misunderstanding and prejudice.[1-3] In fact, medico-moral sexual values woven throughout Western

31

history have contributed to the current stigma experienced by LGBTQIA+ patients today. As such, this chapter will address stigma from a macro and micro level to explain how historical and structural factors influence systemic and interpersonal processes to perpetuate inequality.

HOW HISTORICAL STIGMA HAS SHAPED HEALTHCARE FOR THE LGBTQIA+ COMMUNITY

Due in part to the lack of LGBTQIA+ knowledge, disparities exist between quality of healthcare received by the general population versus that received by the LG-BTQIA+ community. It is important to identify the reasons for this disparity and to examine medicine's historical relationship to sex and gender minorities in order to find ways to remedy this situation. Historical accounts of sexual and gender oppression offer insight into hetero- and cis-normative attitudes and behavior exhibited by many healthcare providers today. Although far from complete, this brief historical context will offer comprehensive insight into how the medical field's roles in constructing stigmatized identities and in shaping past sex and gender patient minority experiences during delivery of healthcare by medical professionals have developed. Moreover, the chapter will also discuss how this collective history may impact expectations and experiences of contemporary provider-patient relationships.

The study, classification, and diagnosis of sex and gender minority groups have precipitated a shift from religious and legal control of "deviant behaviors" through religion and law toward the association of the slightly subtler connotation of social unacceptability via use of medical labeling and diagnosis.[4] Pathologizing identity is one contributor to stigma and all of its harmful manifestations in health care.[5] Ironically, at the same time early researchers had actually worked to end the criminalization of same-sex coupling, psychiatric diagnosis sometimes protected people from criminal punishment.[6] For example, the reframing of the definition of deviance from that of aberrant criminal behavior to one of pathological identity kept some people from incarceration. However, as Foucault[4] suggested, this modified interpretation merely represented a shift in methods used to achieve social control over "deviant" behaviors.

Stigma both arises from and legitimates social stratification, which normalizes the ways in which marginalized individuals remain oppressed by their poorer life circumstances.[7] Erving Goffman,[5] the pioneer of the sociological study of stigma, defines stigma as that which reduces and discredits a person within the social context. While medical theory is not solely responsible for the construction of LGBTQIA+ identities,[8] this historical shift in concern from behavior toward identity caused LGBTQIA+ individuals to be marked with the stigma that has now been causally linked to many health disparities today.[1,5]

In reviewing the history of medicine's (mis)treatment of "deviants," it is important not to lose sight of the importance of agency as expressed by individuals whom we now describe as LGBTQIA+, who have always played a role in the formation of their own identities, actively built community, and engaged in collective resistance.[8] As we will see, it is LGBTQIA+ activism that demanded the *Diagnostic and Statistical Manual of Mental Disorders (DSM®)* be changed,[9] ordered the HIV epidemic to be stemmed,[10] and perpetuated the fight for respectful and informed medical care that continues today.[11] Additionally, while the history here is presented in broad strokes, readers should consider the ways in which interactions with authoritative systems, including that of medicine, are always mediated by intersecting socioeconomic factors beyond gender and sexuality.[12] Indeed, the construction and control of gender and sexuality have a deeply racialized and colonial history that affects healthcare to this day.[13]

EARLY PSYCHIATRY: BIRTH OF HOMOSEXUALITY

Those involved in same-sex behavior in Europe and the United States in the late 1800s and early 1900s were seen as abnormal and deviant.[1] Such views were based on political, religious, and medical motivations for deeming masturbation, same-sex activities, and prostitution as dangerous pursuits. Furthermore, such actions were seen to be damaging to the human body.[14] While some medical texts dating back to the Enlightenment were concerned with presumed health hazards of nonreproductive sex acts, the regulation of sexual deviance was carried out by religious and legal authorities until around 1850.[1] Soon after that, the psychiatric study of sexual minorities began when industrialization, urbanization, and shifts in economic and family structures allowed these groups to carve out social spaces for themselves, while gaining greater public visibility.[6] With psychiatry emerging as a powerful new field, psychiatric explanations of the ills of nonnormative sexuality gained social traction, whereby 19th and 20th century psychiatrists worked to distinguish medical disorders from immoral and illegal behaviors.[1] Subsequently, by viewing nonnormative sexuality through a lens of pathology, negative conceptualizations of sexual minorities were perpetuated by the medical community.[15] For example, early psychiatry commonly viewed acts of sexual deviance as symptoms of "degenerative" hereditary illnesses that led to further degeneracies, such as alcoholism and poverty. Therefore, if an individual participated in sexually deviant behavior, it was thought that future generations would suffer from psychologically tainted genes.[1]

Richard von Krafft-Ebing, who cataloged a wide range of paraphilias and other so-called "abnormal" sexual behaviors in his text *Psychopathia Sexualis* (1998),[16] was one of the early psychiatrists who first pathologized those we would now label as LGBTQIA+. While nonnormative sexual and gender identities have always existed, Krafft-Ebing's medical popularization of the term *homosexual* in the late 1800s introduced a pathological class of sexual subjects to the field of psychiatry.[6] In fact, during the 19th century, physicians were asked to testify against sexual deviants in courts of law.[1] While Krafft-Ebing did not believe that homosexuals should be punished, he pathologized same-sex relations by referring to homosexuality as an incurable illness resulting from a damaged nervous system.[17]

The late 19th and early 20th centuries mark a time of increased scientific inquiry within the fields of psychiatry and sexology through the exploration of the private lives of LGBTQIA+ individuals. Minton[6] reminds us that these people were not uniformly passive recipients of medical research, but rather they inhabited a continuum of varying degrees of agency. Choosing to participate or even conduct their own research as an exercise of self-discovery promoted visibility, increased their chances of finding community, and improved their access to better medical treatment. Even *Psychopathia Sexualis,* which Krafft-Ebing intended as a catalog for medical professionals, ironically gave comfort to many "sexual deviants" who found glimpses of their hidden selves in its pages.[16] Their letters and contributions may have even led Krafft-Ebing to soften his own views.[6]

EARLY SEXOLOGY: NATURAL VARIATION OR ABERRATION?

The field of Sexology was born with the publishing of Magnus Hirschfeld's first issue of the *Journal of Sexology* in 1908.[18] At that time, most sexologists aimed to decriminalize homosexuality by establishing that it had a biological basis in normal human variation. This was the goal of Hirschfeld's predecessor Karl Heinrich Ulrich, whose writings were published between 1864 and 1879.[6] Hirschfeld, a German-born openly gay physician, worked toward achieving sexual freedom for those labeled "perverted" because of their sexual orientation or gender identity.[1] The only treatment he advocated for was one in which physicians helped patients accept their sexual orientation.[6] Later, the scientific evidence that would support such social change was stored at the Institut für Sexualwissenschaft (Institute for Sex Research) in Berlin, a research institute and library created by Hirschfeld in 1919.[19] Sadly, nearly a third of a century later in 1933, the Nazis destroyed the Institute and its contents.[19] The destruction of an institution that contained the largest sexuality library and museum prior to the creation of the Kinsey Institute illustrates the devaluation and social abhorrence that has plagued sexual and gender minorities throughout history.[20]

Dubbed the "Einstein of Sex" by a local paper, Hirschfeld coined the term *transvestite* after studying individuals whose gender expression differed from their assigned sex at birth.[18,21] Hirschfeld's initial description of transvestites is now what is societally considered to be transgender, while the term *transvestite* is considered a subset of cross-dresser.[21] Although the scientific and social understanding of how these terms differ has evolved over time, the systematic and focused research accomplished at the Institute led the way to achieving greater understanding regarding those who now identify as LGBTQIA+.

Havelock Ellis's 1915 work also suggested that homosexuality and atypical gender expression should be seen as normal manifestations of sexuality, rather than as psychopathologic or deviant behavior.[21] However, by the second half of the 19th century, the meanings of "sexual orientation" and "gender identity" collapsed into one another such that they were interchangeably used by the general public to describe degeneration of many kinds, manifesting as the feminization of males and masculinization of females.[1] In *Sexual Inversion*, Havelock Ellis continues this tradition by referring to homosexuality as "inversion."[22] We now recognize Ellis's use of *inversion* as a term that addresses both orientation and gender expression as a conflation of these two concepts. While Ellis eventually went on to introduce the term *eonism* to introduce and articulate the concept of transgender identity as distinct from homosexuality, many people still continue to conflate the two distinct concepts.[23] For example, the legacy of inversion theory, which became quite well known, is that many people view males who display "female qualities" as gay, while in fact they may be heterosexual.

Despite honorable goals of many sexologists and psychiatrists to decriminalize and normalize homosexuality, to some extent these efforts continue to separate and marginalize LGBTQIA+ individuals. This unintended outcome reflects the fact that the medical lens used to classify disease and map out treatments has been also applied to the medical study of gender and sexuality, where it still functions to ultimately pathologize nonnormative sexual identification.[6]

Post-War to Modern Era

The prevailing psychiatric ideology of the mid-20th century (post-Freud) followed Sandor Rodo's 1940 work that claimed that homosexuality was never natural, but was instead the result of a "phobic avoidance of heterosexuality."[21] These ideas led to the inclusion of homosexuality as a medical diagnosis in the *DSM-I* (1952) and *DSM-II* (1968), as well as the barring of open gays and lesbians from the mental health professions.[21] This concept of homosexuality as a mental illness in need of remedy is demonstrated in an educational article written in the 1950s by general practice physician Norman Reider, MD, to his colleagues:

> The general physician, often the first to be consulted by the homosexual, must be prepared to deal at the start with cases of great psychological complexity. Homosexuals are liable to be hostile or paranoid and to present problems bordering on addiction or psychosis. Again, however offensive the behavior, shaming or deriding or reviling has no more place in the treatment of such persons than in the treatment of any other medical condition. (p. 384)[24]

This article not only pathologized and dehumanized homosexuals, but also condescended to them.

Queer theorists and scholars have documented the use of conversion therapy as early as the 1890s, through to the present day.[1] Conversion therapy, typically tied to the post-WWII era of psychoanalysis (post-Freud), was a contentious type of psychotherapy used to cure homosexuality by converting the patient to heterosexuality.[1,15,21,25] Although now viewed as a marginalized form of psychotherapy residing outside of the mainstream of psychiatry, this practice still continues today. The abusive practice of conversion therapy has been perpetuated in the United States for over 100 years. With the goal of coercing a change in people's sexual orientation or gender identity, religious leaders and health practitioners have inflicted techniques ranging from aversion treatments such as inducing nausea, vomiting, or paralysis, to giving electric shocks, to isolation, to talk therapy. Conversion therapy continues to be used in the United States despite waning public support and organized efforts among major mental and medical health associations to ban the practice.[2-5] Healthcare providers working to support minors within the LGBTQIA+ and SGM spectra might be strengthened by legislative as well as professional efforts that advance the effort to end conversion therapy. As of March 2019, 15 states and the District of Columbia have enacted laws banning licensed professionals from using conversion therapy on youth.[6] With continued expansion of these protections, health workers can look forward to a more solid foundation on which to serve LGBTQIA+ and SGM youth.

The skewed understanding of homosexuality as a psychiatric illness requiring treatment persisted until Evelyn Hooker's research demonstrated that gay and heterosexual men had similar mental health.[26] After she received a 6-month grant from the National Institute of Mental Health (NIMH), in 1953 Hooker's research began with a study of both heterosexual and homosexual men. Her results ultimately demonstrated no evidence of increased incidence of psychopathologies in homosexual males versus heterosexual males.[26] Since that time, considerable efforts of gay activists, including a closeted gay psychologist, strove to educate APA members on the effects of stigma. These activist efforts, together with Hooker's research, formed the impetus that prompted the American Psychiatric Association to remove homosexuality as a mental illness from the *Diagnostic and Statistical Manual of Mental Disorders,* Second Edition (*DSM-II*), although this did not occur until 1973.[27,28] Regardless, the diagnosis of homosexuality as a form of mental disease was replaced with a new diagnosis: Sexual Orientation Disturbance.[21] Despite the APA's change to the *DSM* in 1973, the field of psychoanalysis maintained its stance and continued to deny membership to gay and lesbian professionals until as recently as 1991.[9]

Similarly, although the term *Gender Identity Disorder* was removed from the manual prior to the publication of the *DSM-5*, this reference volume continues to pathologize transgender individuals by assigning them the diagnosis of gender dysphoria.[29] While seen as an improvement over the original diagnosis of an identity disorder for many, psychological labeling as "gender dysphoric" does not relate to all transgender narratives and may actually be perceived as degrading by some. That being said, the diagnosis may be helpful to those who utilize insurance to pay for gender-affirming surgeries or treatment.[27,29]

Although the current social and political climate has afforded more freedoms to LGBTQIA+ individuals than they had received during the early 20th century, the demeaning nature of society's view of sex and gender minorities has persisted. Therefore, it is this unwavering public acknowledgment of otherness that continues to make the clinical setting a daunting place for sex and gender minorities.

Modern Legal Consequences

Medicalized policing did not end the legal control of deviant bodies and desires. The pathologizing relationship between medicine and nonreproductive sexual activity has not only led to societal ostracism, but diagnoses have also led to legal ramifications impacting LGBTQIA+ individuals,[30] as engaging in nonreproductive intercourse was frequently punishable by law. For example, sodomy was considered an illegal activity until 2003 in some states in the United States, and those identifying as homosexual lived in fear of being fired, imprisoned, institutionalized, exposed, physically assaulted, and emotionally harassed.[30]

As another example, during the 1940s and early 1950s, the U.S. government likened homosexuality to communism in that both were seen as harmful to society at large.[14] Under McCarthy, homosexuals, as with communists, were seen as potential threats to national security and were fired from government jobs and removed from society.[14] Beginning in 1947 and lasting until 1950, the U.S. government turned down 1,700 applicants for government jobs because they were suspected of being homosexuals, while 420 government employees were fired for the same reason. During this same period, the U.S. military dismissed 4,380 suspected homosexuals from military service. In fact, homosexuality was viewed as so menacing that police officers had the right to enter a person's home if homosexual activity was suspected.[31]

A major turning point in the story of LGBTQIA+ liberation came on June 28th of 1969. Gay bars in New York City functioned as one of the only safe spaces where gay men, lesbians, cross dressers, street hustlers, and queens (individuals who today might identify as transgender women) could congregate and enjoy community. However, these bars were usually operated by the Mafia and they and the police shared the profits of regular pay-offs. Consequently, the police would run regular raids to terrorize patrons under the pretense of enforcing anticross-dressing laws and liquor laws. One of these raids occurred at the Stonewall Inn, a club where homosexuals would congregate, drink alcohol, and socialize.

Stories on how the riots began vary, but accounts center around the arrests of a cross-dressing lesbian and three drag queens as the trigger. This event incited a crowd into a rage that intensified after those who were arrested were forced into a police car. A sudden boiling-over of anger then erupted in the angry crowd, which was no longer willing to quietly accept police oppression, resulting in days of riots. The Stonewall riots were a turning point in politics and of LGBTQIA+ organizational tactics that led to the birth of the gay liberation movement.[32] After that time, support shifted away from the respectability politics of "homophile" organizations, such as the Mattachine Society, to radical leftist politics that spawned what later became the Gay Liberation Front.[33]

Blaming HIV/AIDS on Sexual Deviance

The historical framing of homosexuality was not simply that of sexual desire or sex itself, but that of a dangerous quality that defined the entire personality and moral being of an individual.[4] The "sexual deviant" was then expected to remain repressed, and hidden, or face the justified punitive treatment of state and interpersonal violence, medical neglect and mistreatment, and social and economic exclusion. This classic process of stigmatization served as a mark imposed by people with power (cis- and hetero-normative groups) on those with less power (gender and sexual "deviants").[5] Thus, through stigmatization of gender- and sexually diverse persons as morally deviant subjects, and with the emergence of the HIV/AIDS epidemic in the United States in the early 1980s, an easy hegemony was established in which political representatives and medical professionals refused to acknowledge the presence of the epidemic, particularly in the gay community of the United States, and, when it could no longer be ignored, blamed its spread upon those same marginalized groups, who were seen as "deserving" of their illness resulting from their supposed moral depravity.[34]

Although healthcare professionals are trained to heal the sick, their treatment of patients is often shaped by their own stigmas, with negative consequences for patients. Indeed, "stigmatization of those who are already vulnerable provides the context within which disease spreads, exacerbating morbidity and mortality by erecting barriers between caregivers and those who are sick"[35] (p. 47). In fact, it was not until 2003 that the U.S. Supreme Court ruled that criminalizing homosexual activity was unconstitutional, due to the invasion of privacy (*Lawrence v Texas*[36]). As for the shift in societal efforts framed as the controlling of homosexual acts to the controlling of homosexual identities, the end of sodomy laws led to less overt methods of criminalizing LGBTQIA+ people, especially those who were poor, transgender, and/or Black, Indigenous, people of color (BIPOC).[37] Trans/gender nonconforming people, LGBQ BIPOC, sex workers, and street-involved youth are all still very much criminalized and often victims of police violence. For example, beginning in the 1990s, vague "quality of life" laws were differentially enforced during stop and frisk policing in New York City until these methods were ruled unconstitutional in 2013.[37] Thus, our history built the foundation that continues to support the victimization of these vulnerable populations both inside and outside the healthcare community.

HISTORY'S IMPACT ON LGBTQIA+ BLACK, INDIGENOUS, PEOPLE OF COLOR

The history of clinical care of Black, Indigenous, people of color (BIPOC), particularly African American/Black, Latinx, and Native American patients, has long been problematic in the United States, with racism too often shaping both care and research, even for LGBTQIA+ patients. Many factors affect the care of Black, Indigenous, people of color, resulting in increased exposure to state violence and incarceration and negative treatment outcomes that result from caregiver biases that are still poorly understood. This section will focus on African American/Black, Latinx, and Native American patients. The widespread lack of medical providers of color will also be highlighted.

State Violence Affects Health Outcomes of LGBTQIA+ BIPOC

The increased risk of incarceration, state violence, and resulting poor health outcomes affect African American, Latinx, and Native American populations disproportionately.[38,39] In a seminal 2007 longitudinal study of people who had been incarcerated, the authors concluded that any history of incarceration, regardless of length, increased their chances of developing chronic health issues due to incarceration.[40] Increased health consequences included increased risk of HIV acquisition, with even worse health and other outcomes observed for LGBTQIA+ prisoners.[41] A history of incarceration has been noted as an independent risk factor for HIV, a risk particularly high amongst those in male prisons, especially for African American prisoners.[39,42] Although communities of color commit the same crimes as their white counterparts, the disproportionate arrests and sentencing lengths for incarcerated BIPOC are well-documented. Latinx and African Americans constitute only 29% of the general population, but make up almost double that percentage (57%) of the prison population. Similarly, Native Americans make up 5%, 6%, and 15% of the general population, in Arizona, Montana, and Alaska, respectively, but respectively constitute approximately 10%, 22%, and 38% of the prison population.[39,44] Over half of incarcerated drug offenders (56%) are Black or Latinx, despite reported drug use levels similar to those of whites. Additionally, African Americans are incarcerated at 3.5 times the rates of whites in local jails, which generally lack adequate healthcare resources.[38] Meanwhile, LGBTQIA+ people are at a three-fold higher risk of being targeted by police than are their heterosexual counterparts, resulting in 42.1% of persons in women's prisons identifying as sexual minorities.[44] Moreover, within prisons and jail settings, frequent sex between prisoners increases risk of HIV transmission, due to lack of access to condoms or HIV prevention medications. In addition, there is a marked decrease in access to hormonal care needed by trans patients, even for those patients who had been receiving hormones prior to incarceration. In fact, in a recent study of incarcerated trans women, only one-third of them received needed hormonal therapy while incarcerated.[44]

This lack of care during incarceration—or as *Healthy People 2020* frames it, the failure of prisons in "providing comprehensive health care services during incarceration"[45]—is particularly significant as LGBTQIA+ BIPOC are more likely to be pushed through the school-to-prison-pipeline. Notably, LGBTQIA+ youth only account for 6% of general school population, yet they constitute 15% of the population in juvenile detention, while Black students are subjects of 31% of school-related arrests despite being only 16% of the general population of enrolled school students.[46] Although there is not yet comprehensive data on LGBTQIA+ youth of color with regard to the negative health effects they suffer due to bias and incarceration, more research is needed to comprehensively show the effects of lifetime bias on health outcomes over a lifetime.

This bias in schools and in public spaces is particularly true for trans feminine BIPOC, who are subject to the dangers of underground economy jobs, including over-policing, sexual abuse, and psychological abuse within prison and jail settings.[41,47] The effects of this societal bias cause increased incarceration, mortality, and suicide attempts. Nearly half (47%) of all African American trans people have experienced incarceration, with many experiencing sexual abuse, hormone denial, and extended periods of solitary confinement that have had destructive effects on mental health.[47] Outside of incarceral settings, a rough estimate of the murder rate of trans women due to societal bias is at least 5 to 10 times that of the general population.[48] A 2015 study of 27,715 trans people showed that 26% to 37% of Latinx, American Indian, and Black trans patients avoided medical care due to fear of mistreatment. Additionally, 9% to 10% of all Latinx, American Indian, and Black trans people surveyed had attempted suicide at least once in the last year, much higher than the general population rate of 0.6%.[48,49] These ultimate risks to well-being—incarceration, murder, and suicide—are not often suitably addressed in clinical settings.

Clinical disregard, misunderstanding, and mistreatment have gone hand-in-hand with state violence in communities of color and in LGBTQIA+ communities. In a systematic review of 15 studies on healthcare provider attitudes, medical providers showed low to moderate levels of implicit bias in more than 90% of studies; these biases included seeing patients of color as incapable of getting better, believing that Latinx patients were not capable of taking responsibility for their own health, and thinking that Black patients were less intelligent.[50] "The National Healthcare Disparities Report showed that White patients received better quality of care than Black American, Hispanic, American Indian, and Asian patients."[50] Additionally, a 2019 study conducted in the Midwestern United States showed that poor treatment of trans patients by medical providers resulted from medical provider bias, not from a lack of medical knowledge, as medical providers' hours of trans care education failed to reflect measurable gains in knowledge regarding these patients.[51] In fact, approximately 15% of LGBTQIA+ patients report receiving care of reduced quality due to identity-based discrimination, while 20% report that they avoid clinical care due to fear of discrimination.[52]

Lack of Healthcare Resources and Providers for LGBTQIA+ Communities

In addition to the lack of appropriate healthcare for LGBTQIA+ people, there is also a marked lack of specific community support for LGBTQIA+ BIPOC within the LGBTQIA+ communities. Although highly dense urban areas often have the highest numbers of LGBTQIA+ BIPOC, even large cities such as New York City and San Francisco lack mental health support groups for LGBTQIA+ BIPOC. Such groups are needed to support them while they cope with new social or personal transitions and/or with long-term consequences of sexual variance or hormonal transition.[53-55]

Although many white medical providers build their professional reputations on research and innovation they develop during treatment or study of communities of color, the lack of LGBTQIA+ medical providers that care for Black, Latinx, and Native persons is rarely noted or recognized. Similarly, white medical providers rarely see the influences of their own biases on healthcare delivery and fail to advocate for inclusion of multi-racial spaces to serve communities of color within clinical decision-making and leadership spaces.[56,57] Moreover, medical providers, including those who are LGBTQIA+, too often ignore racist language use by colleagues because it either does not seem racially charged enough or is too bothersome to confront.[57,58]

Mentorship and collaboration from people who benefit most from racism, white people, has historically been extended to other white people, as evidenced by the number of white medical providers (see Figure 3.1; approximately 70% of primary

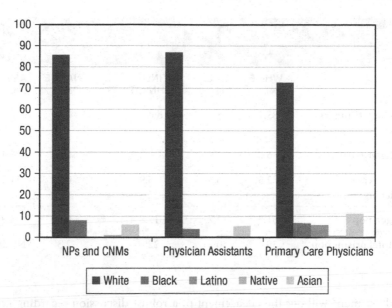

FIGURE 3.1 Racial analysis of providers.
CNMs, certified nurse-midwives; NPs, nurse practitioners.
Sources: Data from Nurse Practitioners & Nurse Midwives. Data USA. 2017. https://datausa.io/profile/
soc/2911XX; The National Commission on Certification of Physician Assistants. 2016 Statistical Profile of
Certified Physician Assistants: An Annual Report of the National Commission on Certification of Physician Assistants. NCCPA; 2017. https://prodcmsstoragesa.blob.core.windows.net/uploads/files/2016Statisti
calProfileofCertifiedPhysicianAssistants.pdf; Xierali IM, Nivet MA. The racial and ethnic composition and
distribution of primary care physicians. *J Health Care Poor Underserved.* 2018;29(1):556–570. doi:10.1353/
hpu.2018.0036

care physicians; 85.7% of nurse practitioners and nurse-midwives; 86.7% of all physician assistants), causing an overall lack of Black, Native, and Latinx medical providers.[59–62] Indeed, mentorship of LGBTQIA+ providers of color is often not recognized
as important for care delivery to LGBTQIA+ communities of color, as many health
centers with LGBTQIA+ BIPOC patients are predominantly staffed by white admin-
istrators. In fact, in healthcare systems in general, 86% of board members and 91%
of CEOs in hospital administration are white and only 11% of executive leadership
in hospitals are people of color.[63] The racial and ethnic health disparities that disen-
franchise LGBTQIA+ BIPOC appear to at least partially result from a lack of representation of this group in healthcare and healthcare administration positions (see
Table 3.1).

Health Inequities Among Black Families— Example of Parental/Infant Mortality

The most stark health inequity in the United States is the well-documented, widely
discussed, and markedly disproportionate rate of morbidity and mortality for Black
gestational parents and their infants.[64] The vast majority of this research has centered

TABLE 3.1 Racial Composition of Clinicians Versus General Population and Prison Population

	WHITE (%)	BLACK (%)	LATINO (ETHNICITY) (%)	NATIVE (%)	ASIAN (%)
Nurse practitioners/midwives	85.7	8	No data	1	6
Physician assistants	86.7	3.9	0.2	0.4	5.4
Primary care physicians	72.5	6.8	5.9	0.7	11.2
% of gen pop	61.3	12.7	17.8	0.9	4.8
% of total prison pop	39	40	22	2.3	No data

around "women" without the engagement of a robust discussion regarding gender identity or expression. For the purposes of this section, we will use the language that the researchers use in describing their findings (i.e., "maternal" morbidity and mortality, which is referring almost exclusively to cisgender women). We acknowledge that there is a paucity of research that examines intersecting experiences of gender identity, gender expression, sexual orientation, and race on parental-child health outcomes.

Outcomes for Black gestational parents and babies are uniformly worse than for White parents on a number of perinatal measures. Black women in the United States are over 50% more likely to have a preterm birth compared to white women, nearly twice as likely to have a low birth weight baby, and have the highest rates of cesarean birth, while white women have the lowest rates.[8-10] In addition, Black women in the United States are three times more likely to die from pregnancy-related causes than are White women[65] and are 60% more likely to develop preeclampsia.[66] Furthermore, the risk appears higher for individuals who are receiving care at institutions that predominantly serve Black patients. Notably, Black women who give birth in such hospitals appear to be at highest risk for mortality and morbidity compared to women giving birth at hospitals that serve a lower percentage of Black women.[64]

The picture of infant mortality is similarly bleak. The U.S. Black infant mortality rate is over twice that of white infant mortality: The rate per 1,000 births is 11.4 for non-Hispanic black and 4.9 for non-Hispanic white infants.[67] As a 2018 article in the *New York Times* points out, today's gap in infant mortality rates between blacks and whites is worse than it was 15 years before slavery ended.[68] This gap persists regardless of education level; infant mortality for Black babies born to college-educated parents is higher than for White babies born to parents with an eighth grade education, while notably 76% of deaths of Black babies appear to be related to low birth weight.[69]

These disparities are due to chronic stressors, institutional racism, and other environmental factors, rather than to genetic factors.[70-72] This is supported by findings that perinatal outcomes for foreign-born Black women are comparable to U.S.-born white women, while U.S.-born Black women continue to have markedly worse outcomes.[73,74] The "weathering hypothesis" was introduced in 1992 after researchers observed that birth outcomes for Black teen mothers were actually better compared to older Black women, suggesting that the cumulative impact of Black individuals' environments had negative consequences for their overall health.[75] The impacts of these stressors on perinatal outcomes for Black families has been documented in a number of ways. Black women who self-reported more racial discrimination were at increased risk of giving birth to infants with very low birthweights.[76] Moreover, there is a 50% increased risk of stillbirth for approximately 21% of all women and 32% of Black women who experience three or more "significant life event" factors during the year prior to the birth.[77] Finally, women of all races who reported one or more life stressor, such as financial, social, or partner-related issues, are significantly more likely to experience postpartum depressive symptoms.[78] When these findings and statistics are considered together, it is clear that pregnancy and birth risks are higher for Black individuals, specifically U.S.-born Black individuals, than for individuals from any other racial or ethnic background.

ECONOMIC INEQUALITY—POVERTY AND HEALTH OUTCOMES

Individuals who live in poverty are more likely to have higher rates of poor health outcomes, including increased obesity, chronic cardiovascular disease, psychological distress, and chronic mental health conditions, such as smoking, postpartum depression, and decreased life expectancy.[79–82] The impacts of poverty on health include limited access to healthy food and lower rates of high school graduation.[83,84]

As is so often the case with intersectional marginalization, LGBTQIA+ individuals are more likely to live in poverty than are others within the general population, and this effect is even greater for women, young people, and African Americans.[85] In 2013, a Pew Research poll found that 39% of LGBT individuals earned $30,000 or less each year, compared to the U.S. average of 28%.[86] For transgender individuals the difference appears to be bleaker; a 2015 survey out of the National Center for Transgender Equality showed that 32% of transgender respondents made less than $10,000 annually, compared to the U.S. average of 23%. Additionally, at the time of the survey, the unemployment rate for transgender individuals was three times higher than for cisgender individuals, and still higher than that of transgender people of color. Notably, one-third of respondents reported that they had experienced homelessness at some point in their lifetimes.[87]

Poverty, Health Insurance, and Access

People living in poverty, as defined as those with incomes at or below 100% of the Federal Poverty Level (FPL), experienced worse access to healthcare, as demonstrated using 18 out of 20 measures of healthcare access, as reported by the Agency for Healthcare Research and Quality. Indeed, people living in poverty were significantly more likely to be without insurance for part or all of the year, with rates of 30.6% and 15.5%, respectively, compared to corresponding rates of 10.2% and 4.2% for high-income individuals who live at 400% or more of the FPL.[88]

WHAT IS THE FEDERAL POVERTY LEVEL (FPL?)

The term Federal Poverty Level (FPL) is a loose term used to describe how the federal government defines poverty. In fact, the federal government does not recognize this term, as it actually uses two measures of poverty: poverty thresholds that are largely used for statistical analyses and poverty guidelines that are used for administrative purposes to determine an individual's or family's eligibility for Medicaid. The 2019 poverty guideline defines poverty for a family of four (in the 48 continuous states and the District of Columbia) as an annual income of $25,750; this is what is often referred to as 100% FPL by nongovernment researchers and advocates. Therefore, any family of four with a combined income of $25,750 or less can be described as living at or below 100% FPL.[11] For Medicaid eligibility, each state has different FPL cutoffs for different populations of people, such as children, pregnant people, parents of young children, and adults who are not parents of young children.

Studies show that LGBTQIA+ individuals in the United States have similar rates of insurance coverage overall as compared to non-LGBTQIA+ populations. However, certain subsets of the population have relatively disproportionate access to care. For example, a 2015 National Health Interview Survey showed that bisexual individuals were significantly less likely to have a single fixed medical care location. Moreover, they were significantly more likely to avoid care due to cost concerns when compared to heterosexual, lesbian, and gay individuals.[89] Other studies have demonstrated that disparities in healthcare access and insurance access also exist for LGBTQIA+ individuals, resulting in their being more likely to have unmet medical needs.[90]

__Medicaid__—Medicaid is a health insurance program which is jointly funded by the states and by the federal government and administered by the states.[14] It is subject to federal regulations, but is administered differently in each state. An example of state differences is "how poor" different groups of people have to be in order to qualify for Medicaid: the federal threshold for pregnant women and children is 148% FPL, but many states have chosen to expand beyond this threshold. However, *nonpregnant adults only have access to Medicaid if their state chose to expand Medicaid with the Affordable Care Act (see below).*

- *Abortion and Medicaid—Another example of state differences in Medicaid administration involves access to abortion care: in 1977, the Hyde Amendment barred federal funds from being used to fund abortions except under limited circumstances; however, some states have decided to allocate state funding towards abortion provision for Medicaid recipients, with some doing this to comply with a court order and others motivated by a limited list of special circumstances.[15]*

***Private Insurance**—Private insurance is health insurance that is not sponsored by the state or federal governments. Private insurance can either be through an individual's place of work as employer-sponsored plans, can be purchased individually, or can be purchased on state or federal "marketplaces" or "exchanges."[16] The exchanges were set up through the Affordable Care Act to provide subsidies to individuals with incomes between 100% and 400% FPL to buy coverage.[17]*

***Affordable Care Act**—This 2010 legislation was created with the goal improving access to better healthcare. The law included subsidies to pay for insurance for people between 100% and 400% FPL, expansion of Medicaid for all adults up to 138% FPL, and systems improvements for the delivery of high-quality healthcare. However, not all states chose to expand their Medicaid programs for all adults,[18] with the highest number of nonadopter states located in the south.[19]*

- *Contraception and the ACA—when the ACA was passed, it was the first law to require that at least one example of all types of contraception (e.g., contraceptive pill, intrauterine device, etonorgestrel implant, etc.) be covered by insurance plans with no cost-sharing. Since that time, several lawsuits and the Trump administration have challenged this provision and have expanded the ability of employers and private educational institutions to decline contraceptive coverage for their employees or students on the basis of claimed religious or moral objections. Litigation is ongoing at the federal and state levels.[19]*

Increased Vulnerability to Poverty of the LGBTQIA+ Population

Studies have suggested that LGBTQIA+ individuals, particularly same-sex married couples, are more vulnerable to poverty compared to different-sex married couples.[91] A study from 2013 showed that 44% of respondents reported "putting off" medical care due to inability to afford services; the same study showed that 4 in 10 uninsured respondents had medical debt and that 48% of the uninsured respondents lived in southern states which had opted out of Medicaid expansion.[92]

Several recent changes have improved access to healthcare for LGBTQIA+ individuals, including the passage of the Affordable Care Act (ACA). The ACA expanded access to health coverage for millions of adults and included specific protections with regard to sexual orientation and gender identity. Rates of uninsured fell by almost half from 2013 to 2016, while rates of LGB individuals covered by Medicaid nearly doubled during this same time period; these changes are roughly equivalent to those experienced by heterosexuals, though gender identity was not assessed in the major study examining these trends.[89] Another change which improved access to health insurance for LGBTQIA+ individuals was the overturning of portions of the Defense of Marriage Act (DOMA) and the 2015 *Obergefell vs. Hodges*[93] ruling that legalized same-sex marriage. These legal changes provided avenues to legally marry a same-sex partner and therefore opening up the possibility for many to obtain health insurance through a spouse.[94]

Coverage of Transgender Services

Many of the health services needed by transgender individuals, such as hormone therapy, counseling, or surgical procedures, are not universally covered by health insurance plans, although there have been improvements made on this front in recent years. As of 2016, Medicare and Federal Employees Health Benefits Program must cover transgender services which are deemed "medically necessary to address a diagnosis of gender dysphoria" including surgical procedures, gender-affirming hormone therapy, and counseling.[92] Medicaid coverage of transgender services varies by state; as of the time of this writing, 19 states ban insurance exclusions for the provision of transgender healthcare; of these, 13 provide transgender inclusive health benefits for state employees.[95] Private insurance plans are not required to cover these services. However, as of 2018 there has been a massive increase in the number of plans that cover transgender services, as shown by the 2018 Human Rights Campaign Corporate Equality Index, which assesses hundreds of businesses, each with over 500 full-time employees; a total of 79% of the evaluated companies offered at least one health insurance plan option that included coverage of short-term leave, counseling, hormone therapy, and visits for hormone monitoring, and for surgical procedures, a number that has increased dramatically from 0% in 2002.[96] For individuals who need any transgender services that are not covered by their insurance, the out-of-pocket costs can be prohibitive, particularly when considering that this population is already at higher risk of living in poverty compared to the general U.S. population.[87]

CULTURAL SAFETY SUMMARY POINTS

Cultural safety for LGBTQIA+ patients, particularly BIPOC patients, must be anchored through an understanding of the historical impacts of exclusion, stigma, and state violence on these populations. Clinical care is not well-informed when patients are seen as homogeneous in population or experience. *Purposeful self-reflection* for providers means seeking out information regarding the ways that oppressed populations of patients have been excluded or treated as abnormal and pathologized; this self-reflection must also include providers' individual roles in perpetuating barriers. In order to *partner* with patients fully, there must be strategic dismantling of exclusive systems barriers through the recognition of and use of our powers as clinicians. For example, providers should actively challenge discriminatory policies within clinics (e.g., the need for "valid" identity documents in order to obtain care, the requirement for which has historically excluded many types of patients—trans, formerly incarcerated, migrant, and refugee patients, to name a few). Clinicians are obliged to engage in systems change to actively combat the historical oppression of LGBTQIA+ communities, and in order to address fuller access to care and healthy communities.

CONCLUSION

- The institution of medicine plays a central role in the history of both creating and perpetuating stigma against LGBTQIA+ patients.
- Classification, diagnosis, and pathologization of identity via the institution of medicine has generated stigma.
- LGBTQIA+ efforts have helped shaped changes in *DSM* classification, governmental responses to the HIV/AIDS crisis, and alterations in policies to further civil rights.
- Intersectional identities often experience heightened stigma and bear the brunt of the burden of systemic oppression.
- *DSM-I* (1952) and *DSM-II* (1968) both included homosexuality as a mental illness and barred open gays and lesbians from the mental health profession. In 1973 the APA removed homosexuality from the *DSM*.
- Conversion therapy has been used to cure homosexuality through "conversion" to heterosexuality.
- Conversion therapy can include such techniques as inducing nausea, vomiting, or paralysis; giving electric shocks; isolating patients; or coercing them through talk therapy. As of March 2019, 15 states and the District of Columbia have banned conversion therapy on youth.

REFERENCES

1. De Block A, Adriaens PR. Pathologizing sexual deviance: a history. *J Sex Res.* 2013;50 (3–4):276–298. doi:10.1080/00224499.2012.738259
2. Harbin A, Beagan B, Goldberg L. Discomfort, judgment, and health care for queers. *J Bioeth Inq.* 2012;9(2):149–160. doi:10.1007/s11673-012-9367-x
3. Mansh M, Garcia G, Lunn MR. From patients to providers: changing the culture in medicine toward sexual and gender minorities. *Acad Med.* 2015;90(5):574–580. doi:10.1097/ACM.0000000000000656

4. Foucault M. *The History of Sexuality*. 1st American ed. Pantheon Books; 1978.
5. Goffman E. *Stigma: Notes on the Management of Spoiled Identity*. 26th pr. Simon & Schuster; 1986.
6. Minton HL. *Departing From Deviance: A History of Homosexual Rights and Emancipatory Science in America*. University of Chicago Press; 2002.
7. Link BG, Phelan JC. Conceptualizing stigma. *Annu Rev Sociol*. 2001;27:363–385. doi:10.1146/annurev.soc.27.1.363
8. Chauncey G. From sexual inversion to homosexuality: medicine and the changing conceptualization of female deviance. *Salmagundi*. 1982;58/59:114–146. https://www.jstor.org/stable/40547567
9. Silverstein C. The implications of removing homosexuality from the *DSM* as a mental disorder. *Arch Sex Behav*. 2009;38(2):161–163. doi:10.1007/s10508-008-9442-x
10. Stockdill BC. *Activism Against AIDS: At the Intersection of Sexuality, Race, Gender, and Class*. Lynne Rienner Publishers; 2003.
11. Sharman Z, ed. *The Remedy: Queer and Trans Voices on Health and Health Care*. Arsenal Pulp Press; 2016.
12. Crenshaw K. Mapping the margins: intersectionality, identity politics, and violence against women of color. *Stanford Law Rev*. 1991;43(6):1241. doi:10.2307/1229039
13. Hankivsky O, Reid C, Cormier R, et al. Exploring the promises of intersectionality for advancing women's health research. *Int J Equity Health*. 2010;9(1):5. doi:10.1186/1475-9276-9-5
14. Johnson CV, Mimiaga MJ, Bradford J. Health care issues among lesbian, gay, bisexual, transgender and intersex (LGBTI) populations in the United States: introduction. *J Homosex*. 2008;54(3):213–224. doi:10.1080/00918360801982025
15. Hammack PL. An integrative paradigm. *Hum Dev*. 2005;48(5):267–290. doi:10.1159/000086872
16. Krafft-Ebing R von, Klaf FS. *Psychopathia Sexualis: With Especial Reference to the Antipathic Sexual Instinct: A Medico-Forensic Study*. Complete English-language ed., 1st Arcade ed. Arcade Pub.: distributed by Little, Brown, and Co; 1998.
17. Savoia P. Sexual science and self-narrative: epistemology and narrative technologies of the self between Krafft-Ebing and Freud. *Hist Human Sci*. 2010;23(5):17–41. doi:10.1177/0952695110375040
18. Bullough VL. Magnus Hirschfeld, an often overlooked pioneer. *Sex Cult*. 2003;7(1):62–72. doi:10.1007/s12119-003-1008-4
19. Amidon KS. Sex on the brain: the rise and fall of German sexual science. *Endeavour*. 2008;32(2):64–69. doi:10.1016/j.endeavour.2008.04.004
20. Bullough VL. Sex will never be the same: the contributions of Alfred C. Kinsey. *Arch Sex Behav*. 2004;33(3):277–286. doi:10.1023/B:ASEB.0000026627.24993.03
21. Drescher J. Queer diagnoses: parallels and contrasts in the history of homosexuality, gender variance, and the diagnostic and statistical manual. *Arch Sex Behav*. 2010;39(2):427–460. doi:10.1007/s10508-009-9531-5
22. Ellis H. *Studies in the Psychology of Sex. Vol 3*. F. A. Davis; 1915.
23. Poteat T, German D, Kerrigan D. Managing uncertainty: a grounded theory of stigma in transgender health care encounters. *Soc Sci Med*. 2013;84:22–29. doi:10.1016/j.socscimed.2013.02.019
24. Reider N. A psychoanalyst replies. *Mon Rev*. 1957;9(8):254. doi:10.14452/MR-009-08-1957-12_3
25. Erickson-Schroth L., ed. *Trans Bodies, Trans Selves: A Resource for the Transgender Community*. Oxford University Press; 2014.

26. Hooker E. The adjustment of the male overt homosexual. *J Proj Tech*. 1957;21(1):18–31. doi:10.1080/08853126.1957.10380742

27. American Psychological Association, ed. *Publication Manual of the American Psychological Association*. 6th ed. APA; 2010.

28. Silverstein C. The implications of removing homosexuality from the *DSM* as a mental disorder. *Arch Sex Behav*. 2009;38(2):161–163. doi:10.1007/s10508-008-9442-x

29. American Psychiatric Association. *Gender Dysphoria*. APA; 2013.

30. Edsall NC. *Toward Stonewall: Homosexuality and Society in the Modern Western World*. University of Virginia Press; 2003. https://muse.jhu.edu/book/16346

31. Andersen R, Fetner T. Economic inequality and intolerance: attitudes toward homosexuality in 35 democracies. *Am J Pol Sci*. 2008;52(4):942–958. doi:10.1111/j.1540-5907.2008.00352.x

32. Carter D. *Stonewall: The Riots That Sparked the Gay Revolution*. Macmillan; 2004.

33. Duberman MB. *Stonewall*. 1st ed. Plume; 1994.

34. Mann JM, Carballo M. AIDS: social, cultural and political aspects overview. *AIDS*. 1989;3(suppl 1):S221–S224. PubMed PMID: 11650419

35. Bayer R, Stuber J. Tobacco control, stigma, and public health: rethinking the relations. *Am J Public Health*. 2006;96(1):47–50. doi:10.2105/AJPH.2005.071886

36. Oyez. *Lawrence v. Texas*. Oyez. n.d. Accessed November 17, 2020. https://www.oyez.org/cases/2002/02-102

37. Mogul JL, Ritchie AJ, Whitlock K. *Queer (in)Justice: The Criminalization of LGBT People in the United States*. Beacon Press; 2012.

38. The Sentencing Project. *Report to the United Nations on Racial Disparities in the U.S. Criminal Justice System*. The Sentencing Project; 2018. https://www.sentencingproject.org/publications/un-report-on-racial-disparities

39. Prison Policy Initiative. *Race and Ethnicity*. PPI. Accessed March 20, 2019. https://www.prisonpolicy.org/research/race_and_ethnicity

40. Harris KM, Halpern CT, Smolen A, et al. The national longitudinal study of adolescent health (Add Health) twin data. *Twin Res Hum Genet*. 2006;9(6):988–997. doi:10.1375/183242706779462787

41. Sandra and Edward Meyer Cancer Center. *Health Conditions That Disproportionately Affect Black Women*. SEMCC; 2017. https://meyercancer.weill.cornell.edu/news/2017-03-30/health-conditions-disproportionately-affect-black-women

42. Valera P, Chang Y, Lian Z. HIV risk inside U.S. prisons: a systematic review of risk reduction interventions conducted in U.S. prisons. *AIDS Care*. 2017;29(8):943–952. doi:10.1080/09540121.2016.1271102

43. Whisnant DE. *All That Is Native and Fine: The Politics of Culture in an American Region*. UNC Press Books; 2018.

44. White Hughto. Creating, reinforcing, and resisting the gender binary: a qualitative study of transgender women's healthcare experiences in sex-segregated jails and prisons. *Int J Prison Health*. 2019;14(2):69–88. https://www.emeraldinsight.com/doi/abs/10.1108/IJPH-02-2017-0011

45. Office of Disease Prevention and Health Promotion. Incarceration. Healthy People 2020. n.d. Accessed November 17, 2020. https://www.healthypeople.gov/2020/topics-objectives/topic/social-determinants-health/interventions-resources/incarceration

46. Massoglia M, Pridemore WA. Incarceration and health. *Annu Rev Sociol*. 2015;41:291–310. doi:10.1146/annurev-soc-073014-112326

47. National Center for Transgender Equality. *A Blueprint for Equality: Prison and Detention Reform*. NCTE; 2012. https://www.transequality.org/sites/default/files/docs/resources/NCTE_Blueprint_for_Equality2012_Prison_Reform.pdf

48. James S, Herman JL, Rankin S, et al. *The Report of the 2015 U.S. Transgender Survey.* NCTE; 2015.

49. Flores AR, Brown TNT, Herman JL. *Race and Ethnicity of Adults Who Identify as Transgender in the United States.* The Williams Institute, UCLA School of Law; 2016. Accessed December 10, 2019. https://williamsinstitute.law.ucla.edu/publications/race -ethnicity-trans-adults-us/

50. Hall EV, Galinsky AD, Phillips KW. Gender profiling: a gendered race perspective on person–position fit. *Pers Soc Psychol Bull.* 2015;41(6):853–868. doi:10.1177/0146167215580779

51. Stroumsa D, Shires DA, Richardson CR, et al. Transphobia rather than education predicts provider knowledge of transgender health care. *Med Educ.* 2019;53(4):398–407. doi:10.1111/medu.13796

52. Powell N, Hibbitts S, Evans M. Gender neutral vaccination against HPV. *BMJ.* 2018;362:k3837. doi:10.1136/bmj.k3837

53. Bertrand M, Kamenica E, Pan J. Gender identity and relative income within households. *Q J Econ.* 2015;130(2):571–614. doi:10.1093/qje/qjv001

54. Lim FA, Brown DV, Justin Kim SM. Addressing health care disparities in the lesbian, gay, bisexual, and transgender population. *Am J Nurs.* 2014;114(6):24–34. doi:10.1097/01 .NAJ.0000450423.89759.36

55. Balsam KF, Molina Y, Beadnell B, et al. Measuring multiple minority stress: the LGBT people of color microaggressions scale. *Cultur Divers Ethnic Minor Psychol.* 2011;17(2):163–174. doi:10.1037/a0023244

56. Moawad FJ, Dellon ES, Achem SR, et al. Effects of race and sex on features of eosinophilic esophagitis. *Clin Gastroenterol Hepatol.* 2016;14(1):23–30. doi:10.1016/j.cgh.2015.08.034

57. Marini S, Crawford K, Morotti A, et al. Association of apolipoprotein E with intracerebral hemorrhage risk by race/ethnicity: a meta-analysis. *JAMA Neurol.* 2019;76(4):480–491. doi:10.1001/jamaneurol.2018.4519

58. Sneider J. Up-and-comer of the month: Geraldine Viswanathan on avoiding racial stereotypes and why "blockers" wouldn't land if it were about boys. *The Tracking Board.* April 3, 2018. http://www.tracking-board.com/up-and -comer-of-the-month-geraldine-viswanathan-on-avoiding-racial-stereotypes-and-why -blockers-wouldnt-land-if-it-were-about-boys

59. Xierali IM, Nivet MA, Gaglioti AH, et al. Increasing family medicine faculty diversity still lags population trends. *J Am Board Fam Med.* 2016; 30(1):100–103. doi:10.3122/ jabfm.2017.01.160211

60. Nurse Practitioners & Nurse Midwives. Data USA. 2016. https://datausa.io/profile/soc/ nurse-practitioners-nurse-midwives

61. The National Commission on Certification of Physician Assistants. *2016 Statistical Profile of Certified Physician Assistants: An Annual Report of the National Commission on Certification of Physician Assistants.* NCCPA; 2017. https://prodcmsstoragesa.blob.core .windows.net/uploads/files/2016StatisticalProfileofCertifiedPhysicianAssistants.pdf

62. The National Commission on Certification of Physician Assistants. *2017 Statistical Profile on Certified Physician Assistants.* NCCPA; 2018. https://www.nccpa.net/news/ 2017-statistical-report-on-certified

63. Bennett WL, Livingston S. The disinformation order: disruptive communication and the decline of democratic institutions. *Eur J Commun.* 2018;33(2):122–139. doi:10.1177/0267323118760317.

64. Howell EA, Egorova N, Balbierz A, et al. Black-white differences in severe maternal morbidity and site of care. *Am J Obstet Gynecol.* 2016;214(1):122.e1–122.e7. doi:10.1016/j .ajog.2015.08.019

65. Creanga AA, Berg CJ, Syverson C, et al. Pregnancy-related mortality in the United States, 2006–2010. *Obstet Gynecol.* 2015;125(1):5. doi:10.1097/AOG.0000000000000564

66. Fingar KR, Mabry-Hernandez I, Ngo-Metzger Q, et al. *Delivery Hospitalizations Involving Preeclampsia and Eclampsia, 2005–2014.* Agency for Healthcare Research and Quality; 2017. Accessed December 10, 2019. https://www.hcup-us.ahrq.gov/reports/statbriefs/sb222-Preeclampsia-Eclampsia-Delivery-Trends.pdf

67. Centers for Disease Control and Prevention. *User Guide to the 2016 Period Linked Birth/Infant Death Public Use File.* Department of Health and Human Services, CDCP, National Center for Health Statistics, Division of Vital Statistics; 2016. ftp://ftp.cdc.gov/pub/Health_Statistics/NCHS/Dataset_Documentation/DVS/periodlinked/LinkPE16Guide.pdf

68. Villarosa L. Why America's black mothers and babies are in a life-or-death crisis. *The New York Times.* April 11, 2018. https://www.nytimes.com/2018/04/11/magazine/black-mothers-babies-death-maternal-mortality.html

69. Schoendorf KC, Hogue CJ, Kleinman JC, et al. Mortality among infants of black as compared with white college-educated parents. *N Engl J Med.* 1992;326(23):1522–1526. doi:10.1056/NEJM199206043262303

70. Burris HH, Lorch SA, Kirpalani H, et al. Racial disparities in preterm birth in USA: a biosensor of physical and social environmental exposures. *Arch Dis Child.* 2019;104(10):931–935. doi:10.1136/archdischild-2018-316486

71. Kramer MR, Hogue CR. What causes racial disparities in very preterm birth? A biosocial perspective. *Epidemiol Rev.* 2009;31(1):84–98. doi:10.1093/ajerev/mxp003

72. Mendez DD, Hogan VK, Culhane JF. Stress during pregnancy: the role of institutional racism. *Stress Health.* 2013;29(4):266–274. doi:10.1002/smi.2462

73. David RJ, Collins JW. Differing birth weight among infants of U.S.-born blacks, African-born blacks, and U.S.-born whites. *N Engl J Med.* 1997;337(17):1209–1214. doi:10.1056/NEJM199710233371706

74. Elo IT, Vang Z, Culhane JF. Variation in birth outcomes by mother's country of birth among non-Hispanic black women in the United States. *Matern Child Health J.* 2014;18(10):2371–2381. doi:10.1007/s10995-014-1477-0

75. Geronimus AT. The weathering hypothesis and the health of African-American women and infants: evidence and speculations. *Ethn Dis.* 1992;2(3):207–221. PubMed PMID: 1467758

76. Collins JW, David RJ, Handler A, et al. Very low birthweight in African American infants: the role of maternal exposure to interpersonal racial discrimination. *Am J Public Health.* 2004;94(12):2132–2138. doi:10.2105/ajph.94.12.2132

77. Hogue CJR, Parker CB, Willinger M, et al. A population-based case-control study of stillbirth: the relationship of significant life events to the racial disparity for African Americans. *Am J Epidemiol.* 2013;177(8):755–767. doi:10.1093/aje/kws381

78. Stone SL, Diop H, Declercq E, et al. Stressful events during pregnancy and postpartum depressive symptoms. *J Womens Health.* 2015;24(5):384–393. doi:10.1089/jwh.2014.4857

79. Levine JA. Poverty and obesity in the U.S. *Diabetes.* 2011;60(11):2667–2668. doi:10.2337/db11-1118

80. Chetty R, Stepner M, Abraham S, et al. The association between income and life expectancy in the United States, 2001–2014. *JAMA.* 2016;315(16):1750–1766. doi:10.1001/jama.2016.4226

81. Blackwell D, Lucas J, Clarke T. *Summary Health Statistics for U.S. Adults: National Health Interview Survey, 2012.* National Center for Health Statistics; Published February 2014. Vital Health Stat Series 10, Number 260. https://www.cdc.gov/nchs/data/series/sr_10/sr10_260.pdf

82. Savitz DA, Stein CR, Ye F, et al. The epidemiology of hospitalized postpartum depression in New York State, 1995–2004. *Ann Epidemiol*. 2011;21(6):399–406. doi:10.1016/j.annepidem.2011.03.003

83. Hilmers A, Hilmers DC, Dave J. Neighborhood disparities in access to healthy foods and their effects on environmental justice. *Am J Public Health*. 2012;102(9): 1644–1654. doi:10.2105/AJPH.2012.300865

84. Centers for Disease Control and Prevention. *CDC Health Disparities and Inequalities Report—United States*. CDCP Morbidity and Mortality Weekly Report; November 22, 2013;62(3). Accessed December 10, 2019. https://www.cdc.gov/mmwr/pdf/other/su6203.pdf

85. Kates J, Ranji U, Beamesderfer A. *Health and Access to Care and Coverage for Lesbian, Gay, Bisexual, and Transgender (LGBT) Individuals in the U.S.* The Henry J Kaiser Family Foundation; Published May 03, 2018. https://www.kff.org/disparities-policy/issue-brief/health-and-access-to-care-and-coverage-for-lesbian-gay-bisexual-and-transgender-individuals-in-the-u-s

86. Pew Research Center. *A Survey of LGBT Americans: Attitudes, Experiences and Values in Changing Times*. PRC; Published June 13, 2013. http://www.pewsocialtrends.org/2013/06/13/a-survey-of-lgbt-americans

87. James SE, Herman JL, Rankin S, et al. *The Report of the 2015 U.S. Transgender Survey*. National Center for Transgender Equality; 2016.

88. Agency for Healthcare Research and Quality. *2017 National Healthcare Quality and Disparities Report*. AHRQ; 2018.

89. Ward BW, Dahlhamer JM, Galinsky AM, et al. *Sexual Orientation and Health Among U.S. Adults: National Health Interview Survey, 2013*. National Health Statistics Report. Centers for Disease Control and Prevention, National Center for Health Statistic; Published July 15, 2014. https://www.cdc.gov/nchs/nhis/sexual_orientation/statistics.htm

90. Buchmueller T, Carpenter CS. Disparities in health insurance coverage, access, and outcomes for individuals in same-sex versus different-sex relationships, 2000–2007. *Am J Public Health*. 2010;100(3):489–495. doi:10.2105/AJPH.2009.160804

91. Badgett MV, Durso LE, Schneebaum A. *New Patterns of Poverty in the Lesbian, Gay, and Bisexual Community*. The Williams Institute; 2013.

92. Durso LE, Baker K, Cray A. *LGBT Communities and the Affordable Care Act: Findings From a National Survey*. Center for American Progress; 2013. www.americanprogress.org/wp-content/uploads/2013/10/LGBT-ACAsurvey-brief1.pdf

93. Oyez. *Obergefell v. Hodges*. Oyez. n.d. Accessed November 17, 2020. https://www.oyez.org/cases/2014/14-556

94. Dawson L, Kates J, Damico A. *The Affordable Care Act and Insurance Coverage Changes by Sexual Orientation*. The Henry J Kaiser Family Foundation; Published January 2018. https://www.kff.org/disparities-policy/issue-brief/the-affordable-care-act-and-insurance-coverage-changes-by-sexual-orientation

95. Human Rights Campaign. *State Maps of Laws & Policies: Transgender Healthcare*. HRC; Published January 15, 2019. https://www.hrc.org/resources/state-maps/transgender-healthcare

96. Human Rights Campaign. *Corporate Equality Index 2020*. HRC; 2018. https://www.hrc.org/campaigns/corporate-equality-index#.Up0UisRDs1J

4

Racial and LGBTQIA+ Microaggressions

Jaymie Campbell Orphanidys, Randi Singer,
and Ronica Mukerjee

LEARNING OBJECTIVES

By the end of this chapter, the reader will be able to:

- Explain how stigma has led to microaggressive behavior.
- Define the term *microaggression* and explain how microaggressions have contributed to health disparity among the LGBTQIA+* patient population.
- Identify commonly used words or phrases that may actually be received as microaggressions.

INTRODUCTION

Although the term *microaggression* has been in existence for over 40 years, research into the phenomenon of microaggressions has greatly increased in the last decade. One of the main reasons for the surge in research and discussion is because of the ongoing issues of oppression that racial, sexual, and gender minorities still face

---

* The authors use the plus sign (+) when writing LGBTQIA+ to encompass additional sexual orientations such as pansexual, asexual, demisexual, and other terms with which we may not be familiar since sexual identity language is constantly evolving. We encourage you to ask your patients what language they use to describe their sexual orientation, and then use that language. It is important to use LGBTQIA+ language instead of the term *homosexual* since homosexual is a clinical term that was used against LGBTQIA+ individuals to diagnose them as mentally ill, and is now outdated and offensive.

despite the gains of LGBTQIA+ and BIPOC (Black, Indigenous, people of color) social movements to decrease biases. Public, visible, and legal segregation of white people and BIPOC—Native American/Indigenous/First Nations/American Indian, African Americans/Blacks/Africans, Latino/a/x, and Asian American/Pacific Islander/Southeast Asian—became illegal when the Civil Rights Act of 1964 passed, and people from the lesbian, gay, bisexual, transgender, and queer (LGBTQIA+) communities fought against police brutality, battled psychopathologization by the American Psychological Association, and achieved marriage equality, which were all rights previously denied to sexual minorities. The explicit and state sanctioned acts of discrimination against racial and sexual minorities are considered macroaggressions because they were publicly visible and affected whole populations of people.[1] Despite the victories won by BIPOC and LGBTQIA+ people, macroaggressions still exist since there are great disparities in healthcare, housing, education, and employment. More so, transgender communities are facing extreme macroaggressions in healthcare and employment. In addition to macroaggressions, racial, sexual, and gender minorities also experience microaggressions defined by Sue et al.[2] as:

> brief and commonplace daily verbal, behavioral, or environmental indignities, whether intentional or unintentional, that communicate hostile, derogatory, or negative racial, gender, sexual-orientation, and religious slights and insults to the target person or group. (p. 271)

In this chapter, the authors define the different categories of microaggressions as they pertain to racial, sexual, and gender minorities and describe examples of microaggressions in sexual and reproductive healthcare.

WHAT IS A MICROAGGRESSION?

Pierce et al.[3] coined the term *microaggression* in 1978 when they analyzed how African American and/or Black people were always represented in commercials as uneducated and inferior to white people. The researchers examined how the subtle, indirect messaging of inferiority impacted the self-esteem of young African American and Black youth, and described the phenomenon as "micro"—meaning subtle— "aggressions"—meaning the underlying, stereotypical, and derogatory messages that were communicated such as African American and/or Black people could not be in commercials as doctors, lawyers, or people in positions of authority, only servants, janitors, and so on.[3] In 2007, Sue et al. expanded the term into a framework, and asserted that microaggressions affect all BIPOC, though in different ways, due to racism and white supremacy.[2] In 2010, Nadal, Rivera, and Corpus applied the framework of racial microaggressions to LGBTQIA+ communities, asserting that LGBTQIA+ communities experience microaggressions because of heterosexism and cissexism or cisnormativity.[4]

Although many dictionary definitions of racism indicate that racism is discrimination from one race to another, those definitions do not acknowledge that there is a distinct power imbalance between white people and BIPOC. Therefore, the authors use the following definition of racism that has been used by many critical race scholars for several decades[5]:

> The systemic subordination of members of targeted racial groups who have relatively little social power in the United States (Blacks, Latino/as, Native Americans, and Asians), by the members of the agent racial group who have relatively more social power (Whites). This subordination is supported by the actions of individuals, cultural norms and values, and the institutional structures and practices of society. (pp. 88–89)

Everyone has prejudices, but not everyone has the privilege to benefit from those prejudices, especially in the realms of healthcare, housing, education, and employment. For this reason, Hoyt[6] summarized the definition of racism simply as "prejudice plus power" (p. 231). Similar to racism, though different in that sexual orientation—who a person is romantically, emotionally, and sexually attracted to—is not outwardly visible like skin color is, heterosexism refers to the power imbalance between people who are attracted to a different gender or gender expression—heterosexual or "straight"—versus someone who is attracted to the same gender or gender expression—lesbian or gay, or someone who is attracted to multiple genders or gender expressions—bisexual or queer. Yarber et al.[7] define *heterosexism* or *heterosexual bias* as "the tendency to see the world in heterosexual terms and to ignore or devalue homosexuality" (p. 572). Heterosexism combines silent judgment with outright bigotry.[8] In addition to its previous definitions, the authors view heterosexism as hetero-assumptiveness; being hetero-assumptive is seeing the world without peripheral vision. In other words, providers assume patients are heterosexual until they deem otherwise despite the fact that most providers do not inquire about sexual orientation, thereby contributing even more to hetero-assumptiveness.

The "T" in LGBTQIA+ refers to transgender—someone whose sex assigned at birth is different from their gender identity. Transgender people and communities face their own specific microaggressions most often from people who are cisgender—someone whose sex assigned at birth is not different from their gender identity. Similar to the power inequities between white people and BIPOC, with heterosexual people and LGBTQIA+ people, there is a power imbalance between cisgender people and transgender people that is referred to as cissexism or cisnormativity. Like heterosexism, cissexism assumes that individuals' external expression of gender, or gender expression, should be congruent with their sex assigned at birth. Any expression or identification of gender that deviates from cis-normative expressions has been and continues to be psychopathologized by the American Psychological Association. Cissexism, as defined by Erickson-Schroth,[9] is a "system of bias in favor of cisgender people, in which people whose gender identities do not match their assigned genders are considered inferior" (p. 612).

Heterosexism and cissexism are deeply ingrained in how society functions and how healthcare services are provided. Many people are unaware of the history and manifestations of racism, heterosexism, and cissexism, which is why Sue et al.[2] established that the "micro" in microaggression does not just mean subtle; it also describes social exchanges from one individual to another that communicate stereotypical, derogatory, and dehumanizing messages about racial and sexual minorities. Sue et al.[2] stated that there are three categories of microaggressions that capture variations in intention underlying the harmful messaging; they are: microassault—intentional, obvious, and usually manifests in offensive humor; microinsult—unintentional, hidden, and the aggressor is usually unaware of the harmful underlying message; and the microinvalidation—intentional if in response to being called out on the harmful message, and unintentional if the harmful invalidation is an isolated event.

IMPLICIT BIAS AND MICROAGGRESSIONS

All individuals develop prejudices and biases that are informed by our experiences of our own culture, other cultures, and how we interpret those experiences. Note: The authors use *prejudice* and *bias* interchangeably since both can be developed from either lived experiences or no experiences but receiving messages from others about their lived experiences; for instance, a person may not have a lived experience of knowing a transgender person, but may have a prejudice or bias against transgender people because of messages they have received from others or from media (TV shows, movies, social media, etc.). Many people are conscious of their explicit biases because those biases most often represent our conscious attitudes, values, and beliefs; however, implicit bias is not only part of our unconscious, it also is enacted automatically.[10,11]

Research shows that many people whose explicit attitudes, values, and beliefs are aligned with social justice actually have implicit biases that are in conflict with their explicit biases.[10] This is one of the main reasons individuals in "helping" professions, such as healthcare, social services, and education, commit microinsults that are unintentional. Microinsults are experienced as painful microaggressions against racial, sexual, and gender minorities. Educating the aggressor about their offensive language often positions racial, sexual, and gender minorities in more danger. For example, individuals who are in need of services may fear or experience their services being impacted negatively if and when they choose to confront their provider. Since microaggressions tend to be more visible to BIPOC and LGBTQIA+ people, the goal of teaching and learning about microaggressions is to make the seemingly invisible more visible to people who have racial, sexual, and gender privilege.[2]

WHY PROVIDERS NEED TO UNDERSTAND MICROAGGRESSIONS

The work of Sue et al.[2] and Nadal et al.[4] support the notion that microaggressions are a very real threat to LGBTQIA+ patients receiving sexual and reproductive healthcare, especially LGBTQIA+ patients of color. For example, with or without realizing it, obstetrical/perinatal healthcare providers commit microassaults, microinsults, and microinvalidations of their childbearing LGBTQIA+ patients. For those who consciously insult or devalue patients through microassaults (i.e., invalidating the lesbian patient attempting conception by inadvertently or purposely reiterating heterosexual childbearing) the path to change may take more than education or training. Education can, however, offer information for when healthcare providers are ready to change behavior and to commit to patient-centered care for all.[12] For those that unconsciously commit microaggressions through microinsults (i.e., implying that a lesbian having difficulty conceiving is not infertile, her partner simply does not have the correct reproductive physiology) and microinvalidations (i.e., not validating that LGBTQIA+ individuals should have equal reproductive access to cisgender, heterosexual people), the authors believe that the awareness gained through education will improve attitudes and intended behavior by reproductively trained HCPs toward their LGBTQIA+ childbearing and childrearing patients.[4] Such basic awareness and knowledge can be gained through trainings focused on LGBTQIA+ patients, particularly in intersectional experiences of LGBTQIA+ patients of color. Use the case that follows to have a collegial dialogue about intentions versus patient experiences. How might the words of Nahda Badpurson impact her patients?

When Nahda has gone to her primary care provider's office for her own care, she believes that she has not needed to worry about being treated respectfully. She is a middle class, white, heterosexual, cisgender married woman, exhibiting several social places of privilege. If staff at the healthcare facility assume that she is heterosexual, it makes her visit seamless.

MEET NAHDA BADPURSON, FNP

- Nahda Badpurson is a 45-year-old cisgender, heterosexual white woman with two live children and a white, cisgender husband.
- Family nurse practitioner and an "ally to LGBTQIA+ people"

Has said the following things while in patient care settings:

- "Sex change operation" instead of "Gender affirming surgery"
- "Which one of you is the mom?" instead of "How does your child refer to you?"
- "He" or "she" instead of the stated correct pronoun of "they"
- "You don't talk like a typical Black person, you are very well spoken" instead of just treating her patient with respect and dignity
- "What are your pet peeves, because I want to be better informed about LGBTQIA+ care?" instead of acknowledging that LGBTQIA+ discrimination in healthcare violates basic human rights

In contrast, when healthcare providers assume patients are heterosexual, for example, and don't even think to ask about sexual orientation or birth control needs, and instead ask about plans for birth control, that is a clear microaggression that patients like Nahda do not worry about. This lack of inclusivity is a microaggression because it quietly invalidates the lives of our patients and sexual minority communities.

THE IMPACT OF MICROAGGRESSIONS ON HEALTH AND WELL-BEING

Racial, sexual orientation, and transgender microaggressions experienced by LGBTQIA+ childbearing patients and LGBTQIA+ childbearing patients of color further contribute to their health disparities. Stress experienced by racial, sexual, and gender minorities due to social stigma has been shown to be directly correlated to their suboptimal emotional health and physical well-being.[13] Stigma, or the widely accepted beliefs that BIPOC are not the norm and LGBTQIA+ people are exhibiting pathology, is one of the main reasons for a specific type of stress experienced by racial and sexual minorities called Minority Stress.[14,15] Minority Stress can lead to increased depression, anxiety, suicidality, self-harm, and substance use, not because of a minority identity, but because of how minorities are viewed and treated in society. Balsam et al.[15] expanded upon Meyer's theory of Minority Stress by establishing the theory of Multiple Minority Stress, which captures the experiences of people who have more than one component of identity that faces discrimination, stigma, and oppression. For instance, a white, cisgender lesbian could experience Minority Stress from being a sexual minority (lesbians are considered sexual minorities), but a Latino, transman who is gay could experience Multiple Minority Stress from being a racial, gender, and sexual minority.[15]

HOW STIGMA LEADS TO HEALTH DISPARITIES

There is a deep and lasting stigma that has historically been associated with being a member of a racial, sexual, or gender minority.[16] It is this stigma that haunts patients who identify outside of what healthcare culture unwittingly reiterates as the white, heterosexual norm.[17] Evidence suggests that LGBTQIA+ patients avoid seeking healthcare services rather than face the possibility of maltreatment and discrimination by a healthcare provider (HCP).[18,19] Many who do seek services commonly avoid full disclosure about their sexual orientation or gender identity while in the care of an HCP, in order to escape maltreatment and misunderstanding.[19] In fact, some individuals have even been denied care by obstetrical and pediatric providers due to their sexual orientation or gender identity.[20,21]

Many HCPs are uncomfortable caring for patients who identify as gay.[22] They may be anxious that they will inadvertently miss something important because they feel unprepared to provide adequate "gay person" care. They may be worried about offending patients by using the wrong terminology, or worse, they may have strong moral opposition to the "LGBTQIA+ lifestyle." Patients are aware of this discomfort and the quality of patient care has been shown to be negatively affected by the healthcare providers' heterosexist and cissexist attitudes and behavior. Most often, the LGBTQIA+ community has responded to the oppression expressed by the medical and legal system by neglecting to seek preventative and routine care.[22-25]

Addressing Health Disparity Issues. Health disparity is defined by the *Healthy People 2020* initiative as "a particular type of health difference that is closely linked with social, economic, and/or environmental disadvantage."[26] Health disparities block marginalized groups of individuals from receiving the care they need because of long-held discrimination against an aspect of their personhood, be it race, sexuality, gender, religion, and so on.[26] HCPs who provide care, including physicians, nurse practitioners, midwives, and nurses, set the stage for inclusion or exclusion since they are in a position of professional power over their patients, and may even be in positions of social power depending on the race, sexual orientation, and gender identity of the provider. Regardless of the identity of the provider, medical education and institutional practices perpetuate systems of oppression such as racism, heterosexism, and cissexism. One way that this is constructed is through the limited options for race, sexual orientation, and gender identity in electronic medical record (EMR) systems. Healthcare disparities are rooted in the knowledge and attitudes of HCPs, which often grow out of racist, heterosexist, and cissexist assumptions that prevail as cultural norms, while systems-based barriers, as simple as our record-taking software, may also perpetuate these disparities.

Challenges Faced by LGBTQIA+ Individuals Seeking Perinatal Care. It is all too easy for perinatal care providers to be focused on their possibly largely heterosexual patient population while ignorant of the daily life challenges faced by LGBTQIA+ communities. Many providers are not aware that in order for lesbians to both become pregnant and maintain legal rights to their child, they may need to go through a multiple-step process. This process includes insemination of the biological parent and, at times, adoption by the nonbiological parent (American Society for Reproductive Medicine [ASRM], 2015, verbal communication). As a result, the couple could incur a large financial hardship.[27] Tiffany Palmer, a family lawyer practicing in Philadelphia, explains why adoption is a necessary evil for any family where there is one biological parent and another parent without genetic ties. Even when both parents' names appear on the birth certificate and the couple is married, Palmer recommends adoption. "The best way to legally protect the couple and the child from a future challenge to parentage is to secure an adoption for the non-genetic parent" (Tiffany Palmer, 2015, verbal communication). Palmer explains that birth certificates are for administrative, rather than legal, purposes. An adoption costs about $2,500 (Tiffany Palmer, 2015, verbal communication).

Whereas reproductive healthcare is covered under heterosexual spousal employment benefits, not all employers extend such benefits to same-sex domestic partners.[28] The Supreme Court decisions to allow consenting adults in any state to marry one another regardless of sexual orientation is a game changer.[29] This decision has great impact in that now spousal health insurance coverage is inclusive of same-sex marriages in each state of the United States.[30] Although the laws had been becoming more inclusive of same-sex marriages, reproductive and fertility coverage within healthcare continues to have restrictive policies to benefit the heterosexual couple trying to conceive.[27] The Affordable Care Act, while supportive of LGBTQIA+ routine medical care by including Pap smears and prostate examinations for all individuals, does not cover assisted reproductive technology (ART). In fact, presently only a quarter of private insurance companies cover infertility treatments.[31] Of that small percentage of insurance companies that do offer financial support for ART, only a few of them extend this coverage to LGBTQIA+ consumers[28,30] through categorization of infertility as medical in nature. Because assisted reproductive technology is state-mandated and can contain language that excludes LGBTQIA+ individuals from coverage (by arguing infertility is structural), LGBTQIA+ couples in need of sperm, ultrasounds, labs, and professional expertise are often on their own medically and financially.[27,32] This institutionalized discrimination is a not-so-subtle form of heterosexism and cissexism, and could be considered macroaggressions. While the nationwide availability of same-sex marriage should increase access to such care, it may take some time to effect real change.

MENTAL HEALTH DISPARITIES EXPERIENCED BY LGBTQIA+ PATIENTS

Lack of culturally safe healthcare services is a common issue plaguing sexual and gender minorities, particularly sexual and gender minority patients of color; this is coupled with significant mental health disparities faced by LGBTQIA+ individuals. For example, lesbian and bisexual women are more likely to be uninsured than are heterosexual women. Although Hooker's[33] research demonstrated that gay-identified men are no more predisposed to psychopathology than heterosexual men, recent research suggests that the stigma associated with being a sexual and gender minority has, in fact, contributed to increased incidences of depression, anxiety, and suicidal ideation for those identifying as LGBTQIA+.[17–19] Gay-identified men are more likely to be diagnosed as having mental illness than their heterosexual counterparts and lesbians are more likely to struggle with alcohol and substance use.[24] Out of the LGBTQIA+ communities, transgender individuals are the most likely to be uninsured and the least likely to access nontransgender-related healthcare services.[24] Increased incidences of mental health diagnoses and substance use are directly correlated with the stigma experienced by LGBTQIA+ patients.[9,34] When people are repeatedly in need of medical attention, housing, and employment, these hardships take an increased toll on physical and mental well-being. It should come as no surprise that a group of oppressed and ostracized individuals would have an increased incidence of depression not because of inherent characteristics of identity, but because of poor societal valuation. The experiences of discrimination and stigma are what leads to mental anguish, Minority Stress, and Multiple Minority Stress. Addressing the stigma experienced by LGBTQIA+ patients and LGBTQIA+ patients of color by educating healthcare providers is the first step toward minimizing health disparities, but more work needs to be done to continue undoing implicit biases and improving care for all patients.

Babymaking, by nature of the sperm and egg requirement, has been seen as a heterosexual, cis-normative privilege.[35] When HCPs assume their patients are heterosexual and cisgender, LGBTQIA+ patients are put in a position that requires them to either explain or be rendered invisible. The responsibility will always fall on the provider to create a culture of patient safety wherein every patient is comfortable with discussing every aspect of their healthcare including uncensored information regarding their own sexual practices. Providers must be clear in their questions to patients that they are not prioritizing cis-normativity or hetero-normativity as baseline or normal, for example, "Do you have a boyfriend or husband?" to a cis-presenting woman.

Many clinicians are hetero-assumptive and cis-normative in their patient care, thereby assuming all individuals are heterosexual and/or cisgender. In most office visits, questions about sexual orientation and gender identity are often absent. This intentional or unintentional elimination of questions directly related to an individual's sexual orientation, gender identity, and relationship is an example of a microaggression.[2,4]

MICROAGGRESSIONS TARGETING TRANS PATIENTS IN SEXUAL AND REPRODUCTIVE HEALTHCARE

Microaggressions would not exist without the stigma within which they are rooted. The stigma associated with identifying oneself as trans/transgender has been shown to correspond not only with intentional avoidance to seek healthcare, but also with rates of suicidal attempts that are significantly higher than the national average.[34,36] What follows is just one example from *Trans Bodies, Trans Selves* and illustrates how microaggressions expressed by a healthcare provider negatively affected one individual's willingness to seek future care.

> I avoid healthcare providers due to my gender identity. I experienced severe discrimination when I identified myself as queer in terms of sexual orientation, and I realize that gender is even less understood.[9]

This type of avoidance due to fear of maltreatment is common among transgender patients as well as many other sexual minorities and BIPOC individuals. Forestalling care may be understandable due to the history and legacy of exclusion experienced by patients who are not white, cishetero-normative within healthcare environments.

Because HCPs are often curious about how a transgender individual may or may not have altered their genitalia, some transgender individuals report unnecessarily long physical examinations.[34] Such a practice can be, for example, humiliating, objectifying, dehumanizing, and/or shaming. Unnecessary genital examination is also sexually assaultive as providers are not performing the examination for legitimate medical concerns. Trans and nonbinary people do at times need pelvic and fertility care and they require knowledgeable support from medical professionals.[37]

Fewer than 35% of healthcare providers ask patients about their sexual orientation or gender identity.[38] It may not be necessary to ask about sexual orientation when providing care but questions about sexual activity are crucial to relevant sexual and reproductive care. That said from a data perspective, decreased sexual orientation disclosure creates a scarcity of data, which may decrease LGBTQIA+ population funding and further understanding of clinical needs as well as healthcare innovation focused on this population.[39]

Though some healthcare providers nearly eliminate sexual orientation and gender identity in their history taking, other healthcare providers tend to be curious and inquisitive about those identifying as LGBTQIA+ and give excessive attention to LGBTQIA+ patient identities and relationships.[32,34] When patients are asked to educate their healthcare provider about their sexual orientation or gender identity, patients' prenatal, intrapartum, or postpartum experience is negatively affected.[40] Since healthcare providers do not ask their heterosexual and cisgender patients to teach them about their sexual practices, LGBTQIA+ patients should not be asked unnecessary invasive questions either. In a recent survey of transgender experiences of discrimination, 50% of participants reported that their HCPs required the transgender patient to explain their gender identity.[34] Such education takes time and focus away from the intended purpose of the medical visit.

Any individual could experience unmet health needs if the healthcare provider focused on their sexuality or gender identity. Lee reiterates this point by intimating that while it is important to take one's sexual orientation into consideration, OB HCPs must be careful to not overly focus on sexual orientation, thereby omitting essential components of care unrelated to sexual orientation or gender identity.[39] To illustrate, in the following circumstance lesbians are being asked to educate and foster knowledge inappropriately:

> I'm not there to educate their staff, so a part of me is sitting there wishing 'please stop asking me about that' and find out why I am having early contractions instead. By all means—acquire the knowledge, but not through the patients. I can come and talk about it later, but not when I am there to have a baby. (p. 2341)[41]

This preoccupation with the patient's sexual orientation, while failing to attend to the patient's pressing health needs, may represent or lead to microaggressions by HCPs.

Implications for Care. Whether subtle or overt, clinician heteronormative and cis-normative attitudes negatively affect the quality of patient care. When patient care suffers, patients lose trust in the healthcare provider. For example, why should the LGBTQIA+ patient follow lifestyle interventions recommended by a homophobic or transphobic healthcare provider? Why should this same patient commit to and show up for appointments when offensive language or ignorant assumptions are likely to reflect the quality of prenatal care? Patients do not want to listen to providers who do not respect them.[42] Why would this be any different for LGBTQIA+ childbearing patients whose healthcare providers demonstrate disrespect through a microaggressive style of care? Heidi, a lesbian mother of two, discusses her response to a microaggressive statement made by a nurse-midwife.

> I personally had a terrible experience with a midwife clinic and ended up going to an OB/GYN for care. Education is sorely needed! It wasn't terrible to the extent that anybody caused me physical harm, but when I asked about their group practice and if we could be sure that whoever attended our birth would not be weird about a 2 mom-family, the midwife responded:
> *'oh, we see all sorts of families here! Fathers who have impregnated their daughters...men in their 40's with teenage partners... nobody is going to judge you!'.*
> I was like, um … did she just compare our family to incest or rape??? We never went back there. But my guess is that the midwives in the clinic probably would have been fine with same-sex families, but they clearly had never had any kind of real conversation about the issue. We went with a lesbian OB/GYN, which was sad because I wanted a water birth!

Patients often reject the recommendations of providers who disrespect them. Specifically, when lesbian OB/GYN patients feel respected and understood by their OB HCPs, they tend to follow through with provider recommendations for preventative care.[43] Although the demographics regarding LGBTQIA+ patients in the general population are not known, these patients number in the millions in the United States; therefore, the disparities in healthcare for LGBTQIA+ patients versus other patients should be urgently addressed.

CULTURAL SAFETY SUMMARY POINTS

Although cultural safety is a process, cultural safety can be achieved with proper patient partnerships and provider self-education. Studies of psychology students suggested that many lack understanding about LGBTQIA+ individuals, which the students believed affected their confidence and ability to work with these populations.[41] The same can be said for clinicians, as they also have not received specific training to prepare them in understanding, communicating with, and caring for these specific populations.[14,25,44]

The heteronormative and cis-normative interactions with healthcare providers described by LGBTQIA+ patients illustrate the lack of HCP cultural responsibility related to the LGBTQIA+ patient. The *Healthy People 2020* initiative addressed the current climate of LGBTQIA+ discrimination by HCPs through its LGBTQIA+-specific recommendations for implementation by the year 2020.[26] Education is necessary in order to improve the knowledge, attitudes, and future behavior of OB HCPs.[33,41] Furthermore, evidence suggests that HCPs would feel more comfortable with fostering clinical relationships with their patients after receiving training focused on LGBTQIA+ inclusion.[45-48] Porter and Krinsky, for example, demonstrated how a single 1-hour training positively affected healthcare providers' self-efficacy when caring for LGBTQIA+ elders.[47] Though Porter and Krinsky addressed best practices in care for elders rather than for pregnant individuals, both types of populations are considered to be vulnerable, regardless of sexual orientation or gender identity.[47] Moreover, sexual and gender minority status adds to their preexisting vulnerability within the healthcare system. While cultural responsibility begins with raising awareness through training and education, true systemic change occurs when new skills and practices are implemented post-training.[47]

CONCLUSION

In conclusion, how the patient experiences a visit can vary according to the language used by the clinician. Lack of respect for race, gender identity, or sexuality can be experienced as biased and not culturally safe, and can reveal a lack of understanding.[49] On the other hand, thoughtful word choice by the healthcare provider can demonstrate openness to alternative family structures.[8] What happens for LGBTQIA+ patients in a healthcare situation may communicate a complete disregard of someone's existence with a gesture or a phrase; a microaggression.[50] They are called micro because they are often subtle and lack conscious intent but can be received as deeply invalidating. An eye roll, offhanded comment, look of disgust, or a discriminating word or gesticulation can all be microaggressions. These microaggressions happen to LGBTQIA+ individuals all of the time when providers use the wrong words and offend both patients and colleagues.

Tips for Addressing Microaggressions

- Microaggressions are social exchanges in which someone directly or indirectly communicates negative, derogatory belief.
- Racial, sexual, and gender microaggressions are pervasive in sexual and reproductive healthcare.
- Include sexual activity, and orientation if relevant, as well as gender identity in history taking, and ask patients about preferred language; then, use that language.
- Take action to receive training and learn how to decrease the frequency of microaggressions and initiate a reparative response.

DISCUSSION QUESTIONS

1. Do you think you have ever been microaggressive?
2. How has this chapter contributed to your understanding of how words or gestures can impact the lives of our patients?

3. If you were Heidi's midwife, and she asked you how you would feel about caring for a two-mom family, how would you answer that question differently?
4. How has stigma contributed to microaggressive behaviors?
5. What other populations deal with microaggressions?

REFERENCES

1. Donovan RA, Galban DJ, Grace RK, et al. Impact of racial macro- and microaggressions in black women's lives: a preliminary analysis. *J Black Psychol.* 2012;39(2):185–196. doi:10.1177/0095798412443259
2. Sue DW, Capodilupo CM, Torino GC, et al. Racial microaggressions in everyday life: implications for clinical practice. *Am Psychol.* 2007;62(4):271–286. doi:10.1037/0003-066X.62.4.271
3. Pierce CM, Carew JV, Pierce-Gonzalez D, et al. An experiment in racism: TV commercials. In: Pierce CM, ed. *Television and Education.* Sage Publications Inc.; 1978.
4. Nadal KL, Rivera DP, Corpus, MJH. Sexual orientation and transgender microaggressions: implications for mental health and counseling. In: Sue DW, ed. *Microaggressions and Marginality: Manifestation, Dynamics, and Impact.* Wiley; 2010:217–240.
5. Gibson PA. Extending the Ally Model of social justice to social work pedagogy. *J Teach Soc Work.* 2014;34(2):199–214. doi:10.1080/08841233.2014.890691
6. Hoyt C Jr. The pedagogy of the meaning of racism: reconciling a discordant discourse. *Social Work.* 2012;57(3):225–234. doi:10.1093/sw/sws009
7. Yarber WL, Sayad BW, Strong B. *Human Sexuality: Diversity in Contemporary America.* 8th ed. McGraw-Hill; 2013.
8. Hyers LL. Alternatives to silence in face-to-face encounters with everyday heterosexism: activism on the interpersonal front. *J Homosex.* 2010;57(4):539–565. doi:10.1080/00918361003608749
9. Erickson-Schroth L, ed. *Trans Bodies, Trans Selves: A Resource for the Transgender Community.* Oxford University Press; 2014.
10. Dovidio JF, Gaertner SE, Kawakami K, et al. Why can't we just get along? Interpersonal biases and interracial distrust. *Cultur Divers Ethnic Minor Psychol.* 2002;8(2):88–102. doi:10.1037/1099-9809.8.2.88
11. van Ryn M, Hardeman R, Phelan SM, et al. Medical school experiences associated with change in implicit racial bias among 3547 students: a medical student CHANGES study report. *J Gen Intern Med.* 2015;30(12):1748–1756. doi:10.1007/s11606-015-3447-7
12. Pro-Change Behavior Systems Inc. The transtheoretical model. Accessed May 15, 2015. http://www.prochange.com/transtheoretical-model-of-behavior-change
13. Institute of Medicine (U.S.), ed. *The Health of Lesbian, Gay, Bisexual, and Transgender People: Building a Foundation for Better Understanding.* National Academies Press; 2011.
14. Meyer IH. Prejudice, social stress, and mental health in lesbian, gay, and bisexual populations: conceptual issues and research evidence. *Psychol Bull.* 2003;129(5):674–697. doi:10.1037/0033-2909.129.5.674
15. Balsam KF, Molina Y, Beadnell B, et al. Measuring multiple minority stress: the LGBT people of color microaggressions scale. *Cultur Divers Ethnic Minor Psychol.* 2011;17(2):163–174. doi:10.1037/a0023244

16. Mansh M, Garcia G, Lunn MR. From patients to providers: changing the culture in medicine toward sexual and gender minorities. *Acad Med.* 2015;90(5):574–580. doi:10.1097/ACM.0000000000000656

17. Lim FA, Brown DV, Justin Kim SM. Addressing health care disparities in the lesbian, gay, bisexual, and transgender population. *Am J Nurs.* 2014;114(6):24–34. doi:10.1097/01. NAJ.0000450423.89759.36

18. Everett BG, Mollborn S. Examining sexual orientation disparities in unmet medical needs among men and women. *Popul Res Policy Rev.* 2014;33(4):553–577. doi:10.1007/s11113-013-9282-9

19. Makadon HJ. Ending LGBT invisibility in health care: the first step in ensuring equitable care. *Cleve Clin J Med.* 2011;78(4):220–224. doi:10.3949/ccjm.78gr.10006

20. Davis VJ. Lesbian health. *Obstet Gynaecol.* 2005;7(2):98–102. doi:10.1576/toag.7.2.098 .27066

21. Grant JM, Mottet L, Tanis J, et al. National Transgender Discrimination Survey report on health and health care. *National Center for Transgender Equality*; 2010. https://cancer-network.org/wp-content/uploads/2017/02/National_Transgender_Discrimination_Survey_Report_on_health_and_health_care.pdf

22. Bonvicini KA, Perlin MJ. The same but different: clinician-patient communication with gay and lesbian patients. *Patient Educ Couns.* 2003;51(2):115–122. doi:10.1016/s0738-3991(02)00189-1

23. Harbin A, Beagan B, Goldberg L. Discomfort, judgment, and health care for queers. *J Bioethical Inq.* 2012;9(2):149–160. doi:10.1007/s11673-012-9367-x

24. Johnson CV, Mimiaga MJ, Bradford J. Health care issues among lesbian, gay, bisexual, transgender and intersex (LGBTI) populations in the United States: introduction. *J Homosex.* 2008;54(3):213–224. doi:10.1080/00918360801982025

25. Poteat T, German D, Kerrigan D. Managing uncertainty: a grounded theory of stigma in transgender health care encounters. *Soc Sci Med.* 2013;84:22–29. doi:10.1016/j. socscimed.2013.02.019

26. Healthy People 2020. Educational and community-based programs. 2018. https://www.healthypeople.gov/2020/topics-objectives/topic/educational-and-community-based-programs

27. American Medical Association. Understanding LGBTQ health issues. Published May 2018. https://www.ama-assn.org/delivering-care/understanding-lgbtq-health-issues#Policy%20on%20LGBTQ%20Health%20Issues

28. American Psychological Medical Association. Resolution on marriage equality for same-sex couples. Accessed April 15, 2019. https://www.apa.org/about/policy/same-sex

29. Isaacson SE. Obergefell v Hodges: the US Supreme Court decides the marriage question. *Oxford J Law Relig.* 2015;4(3):530–535. doi:10.1093/ojlr/rwv047

30. Raifman J, Moscoe E, Austin SB, et al. Association of state laws permitting denial of services to same-sex couples with mental distress in sexual minority adults: a difference-in-difference-in-differences analysis. *JAMA Psychiatry.* 2018;75(7):671–677. doi:10.1001/jamapsychiatry.2018.0757

31. Bitler MP, Schmidt L. Utilization of infertility treatments: the effects of insurance mandates. *Demography.* 2012;49(1):125–149. doi:10.1007/s13524-011-0078-4.

32. Spidsberg BD. Vulnerable and strong—lesbian women encountering maternity care. *J Adv Nurs.* 2007;60(5):478–486. doi:10.1111/j.1365-2648.2007.04439.x

33. Hooker E. The adjustment of the male overt homosexual. *J Project Techn.* 1957;21:18–31. doi:10.1080/08853126.1957.10380742

34. Grant J, Mottet L, Tannis J. Injustice at every turn: a report of the National Transgender Discrimination Survey. *National Center for Transgender Equality*; 2011. https://www .transequality.org/sites/default/files/docs/resources/NTDS_Report.pdf

35. The Ethics Committee of the American Society for Reproductive Medicine. Access to fertility treatment by gays, lesbians, and unmarried persons. *Am Soc Reprod Med Ethics Comm Rep.* 2009;92(4):1190–1193. doi:10.1016/j.fertnstert.2009.07.977

36. Wichinski KA. Providing culturally proficient care for transgender patients. *Nursing.* 2015;45(2):58–63. doi:10.1097/01.NURSE.0000456370.79660.f8

37. Light AD, Obedin-Maliver J, Sevelius JM, et al. Transgender men who experienced pregnancy after female-to-male gender transitioning. *Obstet Gynecol.* 2014;124(6):1120–1127. doi:10.1097/AOG.0000000000000540

38. Nusbaum MRH, Hamilton CD. The proactive sexual health history. *Am Fam Physician.* 2002;66(9):1705–1712. https://www.aafp.org/afp/2002/1101/p1705.html

39. Lee E. Lesbian users of maternity services: appropriate care. *Br J Midwifery.* 2004;12(6):353–358. doi:10.12968/bjom.2004.12.6.13132

40. Röndahl G, Bruhner E, Lindhe J. Heteronormative communication with lesbian families in antenatal care, childbirth and postnatal care. *J Adv Nurs.* 2009;65(11):2337–2344. doi:10.1111/j.1365-2648.2009.05092.x

41. Rondahl G. Students' inadequate knowledge about lesbian, gay, bisexual and transgender persons. *Int J Nurs Educ Scholarsh.* 2009;6(1). doi:10.2202/1548-923X.1718

42. Lacy NL. Why we don't come: patient perceptions on no-shows. *Ann Fam Med.* 2004;2(6):541–545. doi:10.1370/afm.123

43. Hutchinson MK, Thompson AC, Cederbaum JA. Multisystem factors contributing to disparities in preventive health care among lesbian women. *J Obstet Gynecol Neonatal Nurs.* 2006;35(3):393–402. doi:10.1111/j.1552-6909.2006.00054.x

44. Wolfe-Roubatis E, Spatz DL. Transgender men and lactation: what nurses need to know. *MCN Am J Matern Nurs.* 2015;40(1):32–38. doi:10.1097/NMC.0000000000000097

45. Ekundayo OJ, Jones G, Brown A, et al. A brief educational intervention to improve healthcare providers' awareness of child passenger safety. *Int J Pediatr.* 2013;2013:1–5. doi:10.1155/2013/821693

46. Lannon SL. Nursing grand rounds: promoting excellence in nursing. *J Nurses Staff Dev.* 2005;21(5):221–226. doi:10.1097/00124645-200509000-00007

47. Porter KE, Krinsky L. Do LGBT aging trainings effectuate positive change in mainstream elder service providers? *J Homosex.* 2014;61(1):197–216. doi:10.1080/00918369.2013 .835618

48. Reis HT, Clark MS, Gray DJP, et al. Measuring responsiveness in the therapeutic relationship: a patient perspective. *Basic Appl Soc Psychol.* 2008;30(4):339–348. doi:10.1080/01973530802502275

49. Oswald RF, Blume LB, Marks SR. Decentering heteronormativity: a model for family studies. In: Bengtson VL, Acock AC, Allen KR, eds. *Sourcebook of Family Theory and Research.* Sage Publications Inc.; 2005:143–166.

50. Nadal KL. Preventing racial, ethnic, gender, sexual minority, disability, and religious microaggressions: recommendations for promoting positive mental health. *Prev Couns Psychol Theory Res Pract Train.* 2008;2(1):22–28.

5

Trauma-Informed Care

Danielle Boudreau, Ronica Mukerjee, Linda Wesp,
and Lazarus Nance Letcher

LEARNING OBJECTIVES

By the end of this chapter, the reader will be able to:

- Identify an example each of structural, interpersonal, and intra-personal trauma.
- Discuss initial steps a clinician may take to conduct a trauma-informed interview.
- Describe two actions a clinician can take to use a trauma-informed approach during the physical exam.
- List three of the principles used in a trauma-informed approach.

INTRODUCTION

This chapter is intended to provide an overview of a trauma-informed care framework.[1] Trauma-informed care is a specific framework that can be used to avoid re-traumatization, establish safety within healthcare encounters, and build trust between the clinician and patient.[1-3] This chapter is not a comprehensive thesis on the subject, nor is it intended to instruct clinicians in how to diagnose or treat trauma-related disorders; use the references at the back of this chapter for further information on these topics. For the purposes of this book, clinicians working with LGBTQIA+ populations should have a working understanding of trauma-informed care, and be able to integrate simple techniques into their clinical practice.[4] As one of the frameworks used in our approach to writing this book, you will see the threads of trauma-informed care throughout each chapter.

A trauma-informed clinician will begin with recognizing that any individual seeking healthcare arrives with a history of experience with the medical profession.[2] This experience may be from individual encounters, and may also extend back through family and community generations. Whether personal or generational, traumatic experiences are likely to have occurred, especially in patients from marginalized backgrounds, and will influence the experience of the individual seeking healthcare.[1] As clinicians, we are in a position where we can support the process of healing. Our position of power also means we could inflict further trauma. Our goal is to do the former through utilizing a trauma-informed approach.[1,5]

PATIENT STORY

My primary physician has saved my life more than once. On that first visit [to get gender-affirming hormones] I had an entire script memorized to get the prescription I needed and was going to just figure out the dose for the results I wanted on my own. He came in, shook my hand, and looked me in the eye when he asked me questions. When I swallowed my fear and said I was there to start testosterone he said, "Tell me about your gender journey. What are your goals and how do you want us to get you there?" He said words like *nonbinary* and *gender fluid* and I felt my shoulders drop from my ears and my chest open. He got me on a dose lower than what most trans men use, aiming to just stop my period and slowly masculinize my appearance, and he was sure to remind me that testosterone didn't act as birth control. I had no idea that doses could be catered to individual goals. It's an unfortunately rare occurrence for a doctor to know more about trans healthcare than the patient.

I felt like I could open up about my sex history and activity to him. He was so careful in his language and even understanding of polyamory, asking about both mine and my sweetie's testing schedules and safety practices without judgment.

...

I feel like the care I've received with my primary doctor has broken the chain of medical trauma my family has experienced as the descendants of stolen bodies on this stolen land. Not all of my medical experiences have been smooth with my transition. I was harassed and assaulted by my top surgeon, and had no idea what my options were. I opened up about this to my primary doctor and his outrage made me feel validated as well. He walked me through the process of filing complaints (after several intimidating phone calls and meetings [that surgeon] got fired), handled all of my surgical aftercare so I didn't need to see the surgeon ever again, and made sure to notify the rest of the medical community that serves LGBTQIA+ individuals to not trust this individual.

Feeling heard, getting my needs met, and getting to the point of joking with my provider about what my hanky was flagging have all been incredibly healing experiences for me. When we heal ourselves, we heal our ancestors—I hope every Black trans person can have the level of care I've had. All people deserve healing that includes and integrates their whole being—with the cultural competence to understand the barriers to us accessing care or the trauma scaring us away. Healing is our right.

WHAT IS TRAUMA?

Trauma can be defined as the psychological response to an adverse event.[6] Responses to these events may lead to ongoing psychological and emotional distress, including trauma disorders such as posttraumatic stress disorder (PTSD).[4] Types of trauma can be organized into three areas: structural, interpersonal, and intrapersonal trauma.

Structural trauma includes the systematic oppression, marginalization, and microaggressions that impact an individual's daily lived experience in society, as well as macroaggressions such as hate and violence.[7,8] *Interpersonal trauma* includes at least one other person, and may include sexual violence and intimate partner violence.[9–11] And finally, *intrapersonal trauma* is the manifestation of internalized stigma and phobia; these may include physical, psychological, or emotional self-harming behaviors.[5] Individuals seeking healthcare may have experienced some or all of these kinds of trauma in their lifetime.

Structural trauma compounds within communities over the course of generations, and communities are impacted at both the community and individual/biological level.[12] Consider the Tuskegee Syphilis Study, in which white researchers knowingly infected Black men with the disease without their knowledge or consent in order to study the natural history of the infection.[13] Or the forced sterilization of thousands of women of color at multiple points in our country's history, the most recent *legal* occurrence of which happened in Oregon in 1978.[14] Significant mistrust of medical professionals exists among communities of color due to these well-known experiences.[15] Studies are now showing that epigenetic factors are likely to perpetuate stress-mediated health consequences not only to the individual survivors of trauma, but to their offspring for generations to come.[16]

Trauma can also be inherited, though not genetically, by members of communities who do not share biologic ancestry. Although generations of LGBTQIA+ individuals may not be genetically related, the sum of decades of marginalization and targeted violence against LGBTQIA+ people impacts how people navigate today's world safely.[4,10] A Black trans woman does not need to have experienced violence personally in order to be impacted by the knowledge that Black trans women are at higher risk of being a victim of murder,[17] because she has often had to grieve her friends or community members and witness how society responds disrespectfully.

Interpersonal trauma is extremely common among LGBTQIA people and is often related to histories of rejection from parents or caregivers,[18] interpersonal violence, or bullying.[19] Traumatic experiences within healthcare encounters will obviously impact future visits, along with a patient's personal experiences and histories of trauma. For someone with a history of sexual trauma or mistreatment, the idea of a physical exam or even a discussion about sensitive areas or topics may be extremely challenging due to a fear or trauma response. The anatomical areas involved in sexual and reproductive health address physical spaces in people's bodies that may be experienced as the most sensitive and vulnerable, and require disrobing or invasive procedures.[4]

Intrapersonal trauma is an internal stress response that is often a consequence of experiencing external discrimination or messaging about one's sexuality or gender identity being judged as wrong.[20] Examples of intrapersonal trauma include nonsuicidal self-injury or other forms of self-harm that are used in an attempt to manage the pain and distress from exposure to external trauma and marginalization.[21] Internalized homonegativity or transnegativity are maladaptive thought processes that result in behaviors that perpetuate intrapersonal trauma and adverse health outcomes. Disproportionate rates of suicide attempts and self-injury within LGBTQIA+ populations have been associated with previous experiences of family or community rejection, discrimination in the workplace, and gender-based violence.[18,22]

Public health literature has documented the inequities and extent of trauma experienced within LGBTQIA+ communities. The term Minority Stress has been used to describe the cumulative health impacts of marginalization, stigma, and stress associated with being a member of a marginalized community.[20] The personal experience of social stigma has long been associated with poorer physical and mental health outcomes.[19,23–26] We will now review several specific types of trauma experiences that are important for clinicians working with LGBTQIA+ people to understand. These realities shape the daily context within which LGBTQIA+ people live and will impact their experiences as they enter into the healthcare system seeking care and support.

Hate Violence Against LGBTQIA+ Individuals

Instances of trauma are more common for LGBTQIA+ individuals across a broad spectra of circumstances. LGBTQIA+ individuals are at higher risk for experiencing sexual violence.[27] National data from 2016 shows that of the 1,036 hate violence incidents reported from that year, 86% of victims self-identified as LGBQ, and 33% identified as trans or gender expansive. In this same report, 61% of survivors identified as people of color, 15% were undocumented, and 15% reported having a disability—these numbers do *not* include the 49 victims at the Pulse Nightclub shooting in Orlando, Florida, most of whom were reported to be LGBTQIA+ and Latinx. Of these other national incidents, the report found that trans or gender expansive individuals who were also people of color were 3.3 times more likely to experience violence by an ex- or current partner when compared to people who did not hold any of these identities. Additionally, individuals who were under the age of 25 were 4.6 times more likely to experience violence from a relative or family member, compared to older individuals.[28] These findings reinforce what is already well-known in the literature: Risk for violence and trauma is multiplicatively increased for individuals who hold multiple-marginalized identities, such as the intersecting identities of race, class, age, gender, sexuality, and disability.[10]

Interactions With Law Enforcement

The response by law enforcement to traumatic events can contribute to an individual's recovery from a traumatic event and their ability to move toward resilience.[3] The same report written with 2016 data found that 41% of survivors interacted with law enforcement as a result of the hate violence they experienced; 35% said that police were indifferent to their situation, and 31% said that they were hostile. Black survivors were 2.8 times more likely to be recipients of excessive force from law enforcement than nonblack survivors.[28]

These disparate interactions with law enforcement are not new in the 21st century. Accounts of modern-day police brutality within the LGBTQIA+ community—and the LGBTQIA+ community's resilience in combating these injustices—trace back continuously to the notorious Stonewall Riots in New York City in 1968, and the Compton's Cafeteria Riots in San Francisco in 1966.[29,30] In both instances, the LGBTQIA+ community rioted following police raids of known LGBTQIA+-friendly public spaces, and each acted as a local catalyst for activism.

The Medical System and Trauma

Interactions with the medical system may also inflict trauma. For individuals who have AFAB genitalia (e.g., vulvas or vaginas), there is a well-documented history of speculum examinations being performed without consent on patients who were under anesthesia for other nongynecologic procedures, in order to teach medical students.[31] The risks are multiplicative for people in marginalized communities. Chapter 3 on the impact of stigma includes an overview of the history of the Western biomedical community's pathologizing, treatment, and systematic marginalization of LGBTQIA+ individuals. Systematic medical violence against LGBTQIA+ people was openly tolerated—and was legal—for much of modern American history. Examples include the involuntary psychiatric commitment of LGBTQIA+ individuals with permission from either a family member or court judge, the wave of conversion therapy, and forced chemical castration for men who were found to be having sex with men, all of which became common in the postwar era. It was not until 1987 that homosexuality was fully eliminated from the *Diagnostic and Statistical Manual of Mental Disorders* (*DSM®*). The AIDS epidemic of the 1980s and 1990s catalyzed both fiercely anti-gay national sentiment, as well as a powerful rallying of the LGBTQIA+ community, which ultimately improved medical research, leadership, and advocacy in the United States.[27]

In 2010, Lambda Legal released a report that examined medical discrimination against people who were LGBTQIA+ or living with HIV. They used a number of examples of this discrimination: "being refused needed care; health care professionals refusing to touch them or using excessive precautions; health care professionals using harsh or abusive language; being blamed for their health status; or health care professionals being physically rough or abusive" (p. 5).[32] Nearly 56% of LGBQ individuals, 70% of trans or gender expansive individuals, and 63% of people living with HIV reported that they had experienced one or more of those examples of discrimination. One in five trans or gender expansive individuals reported being blamed for their health condition; another fifth reported being the recipient of harsh or abusive language from someone working in the health professional setting. In the majority of categories, individuals who were also people of color or who were low-income reported significantly more instances of discrimination.[32]

These traumatic experiences may or may not lead to ongoing psychological distress, and they are histories that patients will carry with them whenever they enter a healthcare setting. The concept of "sanctuary harm" is one in which harm is inflicted by the very space or setting that is intended to help, protect, and heal.[10] It is crucial for healthcare providers to be mindful of the fact that not all of their patients see the healthcare setting as a place of safety.

WHAT IS TRAUMA-INFORMED CARE?

Adding a trauma-informed lens to clinical care means approaching each individual with the awareness that they may have experienced events that have inflicted trauma on their physical, psychological, emotional, or spiritual selves. A trauma-informed approach attempts to validate past experiences and minimize retraumatization.[5] Trauma-informed care means that the individuals and systems that comprise a healthcare setting actively prioritize patients' needs for safety, respect, and acceptance.[10]

The concept of trauma-informed care originated in the 1980s among providers of substance use and mental health services, who recognized that the majority of their clientele were survivors of some form of victimization.[1] Two of these service providers, psychologists Maxine Harris and Roger D. Fallot, were forerunners in the formation of trauma-informed service models. Since that time, a number of scholars and healthcare providers have developed various trauma-informed models. The body of research and writings on trauma-informed care ranges from guidelines on how to make a system or program trauma-informed to the neurobiology of trauma. The Substance Abuse and Mental Health Services Administration (SAMHSA) has been influential in the development of a trauma-informed care framework. Their definition of a trauma-informed approach, while geared toward programs and systems, is transferrable to individual actions on the part of any clinician:

A program, organization, or system that is trauma-informed: *realizes* the widespread impact of trauma and understands potential paths for recovery; *recognizes* the signs and symptoms of trauma in clients, families, staff, and others involved with the system; *responds* by fully integrating knowledge about trauma into policies, procedures, and practices; and seeks to actively *resist* re-traumatization. (p. 9)[2]

Using a Trauma-Informed Approach

As outlined in the cultural safety framework (Chapter 1), one of a clinician's roles is to support the individual in their healthcare goals. A clinician should not assume that they will fix anyone's history of trauma, or that the only measure of success is when someone tells you that the exam "wasn't that bad." There are six key principles that SAMHSA has outlined as being fundamental to a trauma-informed approach: safety; trustworthiness and transparency; peer support; collaboration and mutuality; empowerment, voice, and choice; and cultural, historical, and gender issues.[2] This is a useful framework to use when contemplating ways in which the healthcare setting and interactions with patients can be reimagined to incorporate a trauma-informed approach. This section will explore ways in which trauma-informed care may shape different aspects of healthcare provision including the intake interview and physical exam. Summary points at the end of the chapter provide examples of how to enact SAMHSA's six principles of a trauma-informed approach.

Intake Interview: When a patient arrives to the healthcare setting for their first encounter with a clinician, the clinician must establish a sense of safety, trust, transparency, and collaboration within a short period of time. It is important to remember that, for some, even walking into a healthcare setting can be triggering, reminding them of past trauma.[5] Remember that a power differential exists between the clinician and patient. Ways to minimize this power differential during a healthcare encounter include actions such as positioning one's body to be at or lower than the patient's eye level, offering to conduct the visit either alone or with a support person, ensuring adequate interpreter services are available, preparing the patient for what the visit will entail, and offering options both for the interview and the physical exam.[33]

An initial step toward providing trauma-informed care is an assessment of the individual's past and present experiences with trauma. A trauma-informed approach encourages care providers to start with the assumption that all individuals have experienced trauma, and to center this as a state of normalcy.[10] There are a number of validated tools with which to assess the presence of ongoing trauma-related stress, including the Primary Care Post Traumatic Stress Disorder Screen (see Supplemental Materials available on Springer Connect; visit connect.springerpub.com/content/book/978-0-8261-6921-1 and access the show supplementary dropdown). This survey includes five questions; if the respondent answers positively to three of them, this suggests trauma-related problems.[34] Another way of identifying trauma-related stress includes watching the patient carefully for signs of a stress response; this may include external behavioral displays such as difficulties with concentration or memory, alterations in mood, or nervous habits.[3] The clinician should remain attentive to other indications of possible trauma history such as overall agitation, eye contact, level of engagement in the visit, body language, and vocal cues.[5] Throughout the interview, the clinician may also gather information that suggests chronic stress or trauma such as changes in sleep, mood, energy level, libido, appetite, or ability to perform activities of daily living; use of substances for mood alteration or stress relief; and physical manifestations such as gastrointestinal complaints, chronic pain, or heart palpitations.[3,33]

Whenever a traumatic event or source of chronic stress has been revealed, the individual's experiences must be validated by the clinician. Remaining calm and recognizing the patient's experience, without pressuring them to talk in great detail, builds trust and understanding. Empathizing with a person's experience can mean simply being present and listening attentively to what a person is sharing. Validation can also take the form of reflecting back what you are hearing, such as "I am hearing that the experience you had in the ED was angering and frustrating."

As the interview progresses, the clinician should preface sensitive questions with the clinical reason why they are asking, and normalize that they ask the same questions to all of their patients. For example, before asking about a sexual history, a clinician may say something like "I ask all of my patients about their sexual activity so that I can make better recommendations about each person's individual sexual health." It should also be made clear to patients that they can decline to answer any question for any reason at any time.[5]

The Physical Exam: Ideally, the entire introductory interview was conducted before the patient was asked to remove any items of clothing necessary for the physical exam. Prior to initiation of the physical exam, the details of the exam and the rationale behind each piece should be discussed with the patient. Similar to the approach for sensitive questions during the interview, it should also be made clear to patients that they can decline any portion of the physical exam. For any physical exam, the patient should be offered options to perform as much themselves as is possible: for example, this may include moving aside clothing or the drape for each part of the exam, collecting self-swabs, or self-insertion of the speculum.

Throughout the exam, the clinician should explain the reason for the next step, ask for permission before performing each section of the physical exam, describe the physical sensations that may occur (e.g., "You may notice a gagging sensation during the throat swab"), and describe the visual or auditory stimuli that may occur (e.g., "You will hear the rattling of the drawer while I get the speculum for the next part of the exam"). It is also important to offer options for verbal and nonverbal cues that the patient can use to signal that they are done with the exam, need a break, or need an adjustment.[33]

A more detailed discussion of trauma-informed chest and pelvic exams is included in Chapter 10 on sexual healthcare for LGBTQIA+ individuals.

CLINICIAN VOICES—MIDWIFERY STUDENT

I attended a conference one year where the topic of trauma-informed pelvic care came up. We were discussing how to provide sensitive pelvic exams, and I thought of a scenario that at the time I thought was revolutionary, if only because I had performed perhaps a couple dozen pelvic examinations at that point. I asked the group: "But what if the patient tells you to keep going with the exam, but everything in their body language is telling you to stop, like they are reliving their trauma all over again?" The resounding answer from the group was: *keep going*. Listen to your patient. It may be that their goals are to be screened for cervical cancer, and it may be that their body will respond in ways that will make you, the clinician, uncomfortable. But of course, it is not about you.

THE ROLE OF IMPLICIT BIAS

Implicit bias has already been mentioned in this book, and deserves mention again here in this chapter as we now understand more about how trauma impacts our patients and the importance of creating healthcare encounters where re-traumatization does not occur.[35] As you may recall, implicit bias is the unconscious stereotypes and associations held about a particular group of people. Healthcare providers are not immune from implicit bias, and it has been shown to impact care of LGBTQIA+ populations in addition to racial and ethnic minorities[36–38] even among clinicians who are members of marginalized groups themselves.[35] Implicit bias among clinicians is a potential source of re-traumatization for patients and must be addressed.[5] Clinicians can start to become mindful of their own implicit bias by noticing when they feel uncertain,[37,39] observing when they have a "gut reaction" to something that occurs during a patient encounter, and being willing to reschedule a follow-up visit with the patient if they find they need additional time to research a particular issue, rather than acting from a place of reactivity.[5] Recognizing and addressing our implicit bias takes attentiveness and practice. See the box that follows for some tools you can use to evaluate and reduce your own implicit bias.

IT TAKES PRACTICE!

Overcoming implicit bias takes practice. There are a number of tools that have been designed in order to help clinicians identify and overcome their own implicit biases. Take a few moments to check out the following tools and resources available to you.

- National LGBT Health Education Center's Case Scenarios: www.lgbthealtheducation.org/publication/learning-to-address-implicit-bias-towards-lgbtq-patients-case-scenarios. This publication guides you through various clinical scenarios with tips and tools for communication and advocacy with LGBTQIA+ populations in clinical settings.
- Harvard Implicit Association Test: https://implicit.harvard.edu/implicit/takeatest.html. Project Implicit has created a variety of self-tests to bring awareness to the thoughts and feelings that are outside of our conscious awareness and may impact our actions implicitly. You can take tests that evaluate your own individual levels of implicit bias regarding sexuality, as well as race, disability, age, weight, or various other social categories.

CULTURAL SAFETY SUMMARY POINTS

What follows are examples of how clinicians may consider incorporating SAMHSA's six key principles of trauma-informed care into their practice.

Safety

- Assume that everyone has a history of trauma.
- Allow the patient to lead the way.
- Do not re-traumatize.

Trustworthiness and Transparency

- Disclose why you are asking certain questions.
- Explain what you will do with the information they disclose.

Peer Support

- Get to know your community and the resources within it.
- Always ask permission before connecting them with an individual or organization.

Collaboration and Mutuality

- Decide on the shared vocabulary that you will both use to conduct the visit.
- Agree upon shared goals or desired outcomes.
- Offer options, such as how to collect a sample or what area they would like to focus on in the visit today.

Empowerment, Voice, and Choice

- Ask questions.
- Model verbal and nonverbal cues the patient may use to decline to answer a question or decline a part of the exam.
- Respect their boundaries.
- Use reflective language, maintain neutrality.
- Offer choices of what to focus on for each visit, which parts of the exam to conduct, and how to achieve different aspects of the physical examination.

Cultural, Historical, and Gender Issues

- Pay attention to multiple marginalities.
- Acknowledge that this may (or may not) be a difficult experience for them.

CONCLUSION: MOVING TOWARD RESILIENCE

An individual's ability to heal from traumatic events and move toward active recognition of their own resilience depends on a multitude of factors: when the event occurred, how often it occurred and how long it lasted, how severe it was, and what their developmental or intellectual capacity for understanding was at the time of the event. It also is impacted by the messages the individual has received from others: were they listened to, validated, blamed, supported, or believed? What are the messages, norms, and values that they internalized from the culture in which they were raised?[3] While a clinician cannot change those events that have already occurred, they may be able to aid the individual in identifying resources that will aid in their future recovery. These resources include already-existing networks of social and familial support, legal protections and resources, access to affirming physical and mental health care, and management of other personal health and well-being.[3] The steps included in providing a trauma-informed healthcare visit can also promote resilience by valuing empowerment, engagement, and collaboration.[2]

DISCUSSION QUESTIONS

1. What are the barriers you might anticipate in implementing a trauma-informed framework within the healthcare system you work in?
2. How would you go about practicing the language you might use in a trauma-informed office visit?
3. What are ways in which you might promote resilience within the specific communities that you serve?

REFERENCES

1. Sciolla A. An overview of trauma-informed care. In: Eckstrand KL, Potter J, eds. *Trauma, Resilience, and Health Promotion in LGBT Patients: What Every Healthcare Provider Should Know.* Springer International Publishing; 2017:165–182. https://www.springer.com/us/book/9783319545073
2. Substance Abuse and Mental Health Services Administration. SAMHSA's concept of trauma and guidance for a trauma-informed approach. 2014. https://store.samhsa.gov/product/SAMHSA-s-Concept-of-Trauma-and-Guidance-for-a-Trauma-Informed-Approach/SMA14-4884.html
3. Kudler B, Presley C, Savage M. Trauma-informed care: addressing mental health risk factors. Oral presentation at: Advancing Excellence in Transgender Health; October, 2015; Boston, MA.
4. Alessi E, Martin J. Intersection of trauma and identity. In: Eckstrand KL, Potter J, eds. *Trauma, Resilience, and Health Promotion in LGBT Patients: What Every Healthcare Provider Should Know.* Springer International Publishing; 2017:3–14. https://www.springer.com/us/book/9783319545073

5. Poteat T, Singh A. Conceptualizing trauma in clinical settings: iatrogenic harm and bias. In: Eckstrand KL, Potter J, eds. *Trauma, Resilience, and Health Promotion in LGBT Patients: What Every Healthcare Provider Should Know.* Springer International Publishing; 2017:25–34. https://www.springer.com/us/book/9783319545073

6. American Psychological Association. Trauma. Accessed April 13, 2019. https://www.apa.org/topics/trauma

7. Center for Health Equity Research Chicago. What is structural violence? 2018. http://www.cherchicago.org/about/structuralviolence

8. Basnyat I. Structural violence in health care: lived experience of street-based female commercial sex workers in Kathmandu. *Qual Health Res.* 2017;27(2):191–203. doi:10.1177/1049732315601665

9. Ma PHX, Chan ZCY, Loke AY. The socio-ecological model approach to understanding barriers and facilitators to the accessing of health services by sex workers: a systematic review. *AIDS Behav.* 2017;21(8):2412–2438. doi:10.1007/s10461-017-1818-2

10. Miller E, Goodman L, Thomas K, et al. Trauma-informed approaches for LGBTQ* survivors of intimate partner violence: a review of literature and a set of practice observations. The GLBTQ Domestic Violence Project; 2016. http://www.nationalcenterdvtraumamh.org/publications-products/trauma-informed-approaches-for-lgbqt-survivors-of-intimate-partner-violence-a-review-of-literature-and-a-set-of-practice-observations

11. Hyers LL. Alternatives to silence in face-to-face encounters with everyday heterosexism: activism on the interpersonal front. *J Homosex.* 2010;57(4):539–565. doi:10.1080/00918361003608749

12. Yehuda R, Lehrner A. Intergenerational transmission of trauma effects: putative role of epigenetic mechanisms. *World Psychiatry.* 2018;17(3):243–257. doi:10.1002/wps.20568

13. Smith SL. Neither victim nor villain: Nurse Eunice Rivers, the Tuskegee Syphilis Experiment, and Public Health Work. *J Women's Hist.* 1996;8(1):95–113. doi:10.13016/irzb-q8li

14. Rutecki G. Forced sterilization of Native Americans: later twentieth century cooperation with national eugenic policies? *Ethics Med.* 2011;27(1):33–42.

15. Washington HA. *Medical Apartheid: The Dark History of Medical Experimentation on Black Americans From Colonial Times to the Present.* 1st ed. Harlem Moon; 2006.

16. Brockie TN, Heinzelmann M, Gill J. A framework to examine the role of epigenetics in health disparities among Native Americans. *Nurs Res Pract.* 2013;2013:1–9. doi:10.1155/2013/410395

17. Dinno A. Homicide rates of transgender individuals in the United States: 2010–2014. *Am J Public Health.* 2017;107(9):1441–1447. doi:10.2105/AJPH.2017.303878

18. Klein A, Golub SA. Family rejection as a predictor of suicide attempts and substance misuse among transgender and gender nonconforming adults. *LGBT Health.* 2016;3(3):193–199. doi:10.1089/lgbt.2015.0111

19. Gamarel KE, Reisner SL, Laurenceau J-P, et al. Gender minority stress, mental health, and relationship quality: a dyadic investigation of transgender women and their cisgender male partners. *J Fam Psychol.* 2014;28(4):437–447. doi:10.1037/a0037171

20. Meyer IH. Prejudice, social stress, and mental health in lesbian, gay, and bisexual populations: conceptual issues and research evidence. *Psychol Bull.* 2003;129(5):674–697. doi:10.1037/0033-2909.129.5.674

21. Claes L, Bouman WP, Witcomb G, et al. Non-suicidal self-injury in trans people: associations with psychological symptoms, victimization, interpersonal functioning, and perceived social support. *J Sex Med.* 2015;12(1):168–179. doi:10.1111/jsm.12711

22. James S, Herman JL, Rankin S, et al. *The Report of the 2015 U.S. Transgender Survey.* National Center for Transgender Equality; 2015.

23. Huebner DM, Davis MC. Perceived antigay discrimination and physical health outcomes. *Health Psychol.* 2007;26(5):627–634. doi:10.1037/0278-6133.26.5.627

24. Meyer IH. Minority stress and mental health in gay men. *J Health Soc Behav.* 1995;36(1):38–56. https://www.jstor.org/stable/2137286

25. Lewis RJ, Derlega VJ, Clarke EG, et al. Stigma consciousness, social constraints, and lesbian well-being. *J Couns Psychol.* 2006;53(1):48–56. doi:10.1037/0022-0167.53.1.48

26. Bockting WO, Miner MH, Swinburne Romine RE, et al. Stigma, mental health, and resilience in an online sample of the US transgender population. *Am J Public Health.* 2013;103(5):943–951. doi:10.2105/AJPH.2013.301241

27. Shapiro S, Powell T. Medical intervention and LGBT people: a brief history. In: Eckstrand KL, Potter J, eds. *Trauma, Resilience, and Health Promotion in LGBT Patients: What Every Healthcare Provider Should Know.* Springer International Publishing; 2017:15–24. https://www.springer.com/us/book/9783319545073

28. Waters E. *Lesbian, Gay, Bisexual, Transgender, Queer, and HIV-Affected Hate Violence in 2016.* New York City Anti-Violence Project Inc.; 2017.

29. Kuhn B. *Gay Power!: The Stonewall Riots and the Gay Rights Movement, 1969.* Twenty-First Century Books; 2011. https://lernerbooks.com/shop/show/12145

30. Feinberg L. *Stone Butch Blues.* Firebrand Books; 1993. https://www.abebooks.com/first-edition/STONE-BUTCH-BLUES-Leslie-Feinberg-Firebrand/17130429069/bd

31. Wilson RF. Unauthorized practice: teaching pelvic examination on women under anesthesia. *J Am Med Womens Assoc 1972.* 2003;58(4):217–220; discussion 221–222. PMID: 14640251.

32. Lambda Legal. When health care isn't caring. 2010. https://www.lambdalegal.org/health-care-report

33. Ravi A, Little V. Providing trauma-informed care. *Am Fam Physician.* 2017;95(10):655–657. https://www.aafp.org/afp/2017/0515/p655.html

34. Prins A, Bovin MJ, Smolenski DJ, et al. The primary care PTSD screen for *DSM-5* (PC-PTSD-5): development and evaluation within a veteran primary care sample. *J Gen Intern Med.* 2016;31(10):1206–1211. doi:10.1007/s11606-016-3703-5

35. Sabin JA, Riskind RG, Nosek BA. Health care providers' implicit and explicit attitudes toward lesbian women and gay men. *Am J Public Health.* 2015;105(9):1831–1841. doi:10.2105/AJPH.2015.302631

36. Poteat T, German D, Kerrigan D. Managing uncertainty: a grounded theory of stigma in transgender health care encounters. *Soc Sci Med 1982.* 2013;84:22–29. doi:10.1016/j.socscimed.2013.02.019

37. Dorsen C. An integrative review of nurse attitudes towards lesbian, gay, bisexual, and transgender patients. *Can J Nurs Res.* 2012;44(3):18–43. PMID: 23156190.

38. Carabez R, Pellegrini M, Mankovitz A, et al. Does your organization use gender inclusive forms? Nurses' confusion about trans* terminology. *J Clin Nurs.* 2015;24(21–22):3306–3317. doi:10.1111/jocn.12942

39. Poteat T, Wirtz AL, Radix A, et al. HIV risk and preventive interventions in transgender women sex workers. *Lancet.* 2015;385(9964):274–286. doi:10.1016/S0140-6736(14)60833-3

II

People and Identities

6

Queerness and Sexualities

Ronica Mukerjee, D'hana Perry, and Linda Wesp

LEARNING OBJECTIVES

By the end of this chapter, the reader will be able to:

- Understand the various ways people use the term *queer* regarding their sexualities.*
- Explore ways to work with queer patients in clinical environments.
- Describe some recommendations in caring for queer-identified patients.

INTRODUCTION

In this introductory chapter to Part II of this book, the People and Identities section, we begin with exploring queerness and sexuality. Understanding sexual identities and what they may mean for our patients helps us to elucidate provision of care for those individuals who identify outside of the classically heterosexual definition of sexuality. Definitions and historical contexts of queerness are vibrantly variable.[1,2] This chapter is not meant to be a comprehensive primer on queerness, which is consistently—and occasionally contentiously—shifting. Queerness is complex, and carries a diversity of meanings to its many constituents. Because of its variability, attempts to comprehensively define the concept will inevitably omit certain groups and individuals who identify as queer.[3] As such, this chapter will offer greater knowledge without claiming comprehensiveness.

---

* For information about queerness and trans identity, please see Chapter 9: Gender Identity. For more information about asexuality and queerness, see Chapter 7: Asexual Patient Care. For discussion of overlap between intersex people and queer identities, see Chapter 8: Intersex Patient Care.

Queer and *queerness* are considered to be umbrella terms used to express fluid identities and orientations and are often used interchangeably with "LGBTQIA+" identities.[4] When working with queer-identified patients, it is important to understand that queer identities are multidimensional and are often inclusive of many sexual orientations, gender identities, gender expressions, and sexual behaviors.[5] Queerness, however, is not solely applicable to sexuality or gender: 'queer' also encompasses cultural and political affiliations that will often, but not always, set queer-identified people apart from mainstream gays and lesbians. This chapter will focus less on political aspects of queerness, but rather on queerness and its relationship to sexuality.[1,2]

There are many sexual identities that exist within and outside of the queer framework. Some general categories to describe sexual identities that overlap with other categories include lesbian, gay, bisexual, pansexual and/or queer (see Table 6.1). Cultures not represented well by United States LGBTQIA+ demographics may use alternative terms; for example, the term *kothi* to indicate South Asian MAAB (male assigned at birth) people who have sex with MAAB people while, at times, presenting with a gender expression that is feminine of center.[6] *Nongay'ndoda* is a Xhosa (South African) term, at times pejorative but also gaining acceptance among FAAB (female assigned at birth) individuals who are masculine of center and are attracted to/sexually active with other FAAB people.[7]

TABLE 6.1 Descriptors of Some Sexual Identities in the United States

IDENTITY	BRIEF DESCRIPTION
Lesbian	Woman/femmes (including e.g., trans women/femmes/butch women) who identify with primarily having sex with women
Gay	Refers to men/mascs (including e.g., trans men/mascs/femme gay men) who are primarily attracted to men
Bisexual	Individuals who are attracted to more than one gender
Pansexual	Individuals whose attractions are not limited by biological sex or gender
Queer	Nonheterosexual sexual identity; can be fluid and can be a political identity
Same Gender Loving/ Same Gender Attracted (SGL/SGA)	Sometimes used by African American individuals to express sexual orientation, eschewing European definitions. Same gender attracted is for individuals who are speaking to attraction only
MSM	Men who have sex with men; this term includes trans masculine patients. Sometimes trans feminine patients are inappropriately lumped into this category in research settings

Despite the longevity of some of the available terms for sexual identity, further description is needed to more clearly understand the sexual identities that patients and LGBTQIA+ populations may hold. The traditional definitions of sexuality were often steeped in de facto assumptions of sexual activities while also failing to be inclusive of people who rejected, did not feel inside of, or held identities that did not fall into the neat boxes of "gay" and "straight." Queer as a label or identity can feel ambiguous and undefined to some, and correct in its lack of assumptions for others. There may be those within the LGBTQIA+ community who still see *queer* as a historically pejorative term and, in an effort to preserve their own identities, distance themselves intentionally from queer-identified communities.[5]

QUEERNESS AS SEXUAL IDENTITY

Queer sexual identity can be adopted by people who express their sexualities in a variety of ways, including not being typically sexual at all (see Chapter 7). The term can be used in conjunction with "lesbian," for example, where individuals might identify as both queer and a lesbian or, less frequently, as a *queer lesbian*. The same can be said about other terms like *pansexual*, which can similarly be coupled with queer (aka *queer and pansexual*), and, less commonly, as *queer pansexual*. Queerness can be adopted by those who feel that their sexualities are not properly captured by the singular terms, such as *gay, lesbian,* or *bisexual*. Individuals who are queer may also identify as lesbian, gay, trans, asexual or a combination of those intersecting identities.[1,2]

Some examples of how people may describe their identity:

- Xavier is a queer pansexual genderqueer person.
- Radhika is a nonbinary lesbian who identifies as queer.
- Estrella is a queer gay hijra.
- Kofi is an asexual bisexual agender person who identifies as queer.
- Jen is a polyamorous queer cisgender female.
- Emmett is a queer trans man.

Queerness can express a discrete layer of someone's sexual identity without necessarily giving information about their sexual behavior—which could potentially range from not sexually active (asexual) to highly sexual, relatively cis-heterosexual to relatively cis-homosexual. Some trans people may also identify as both heterosexual and queer because they see their attractions as cross-gender attractions but also see themselves as part of queer community. To be very specific, **people of any gender, including agender people, can have sex with any other gender of person without it affecting their personal sexual identity, including their identity as queer.** In other words, an identity label, such as queer, describes important aspects of a person but is not prescriptive of their behavior. For example, a trans woman who only has sex with trans men identifies as lesbian and queer, while having sex that involves penile-vaginal penetrative sex.

Aspects of sexual identity can include kink practices, which encompass a wide variety of sexual or sexualized practices, desires, and identities, alongside sexual fetishism and bondage, discipline, domination, and submission as well as sadism and masochism (BDSM) practices. This broad spectrum of sexual behaviors may exist within a variety of queer communities and relationships. Individuals within kink communities often identify their sexual practices as distinct from mainstream heterosexuality even though there might be some overlap with classic heterosexual practices. While not all people who participate in kink practices identify as queer, kink communities can be queer-friendly spaces, and are more likely to contain people who express both sexual and gender variance.[8,9]

FURTHER INFORMATION ON KINK/BDSM

- **Recommended Reading on BDSM for Healthcare Providers:** www.chicagodungeonrentals.com/wp-content/uploads/2016/04/Resources-Handout-Compassionate-Care-for-Kinky-People.pdf
- **Kink Therapy Certification Institute:** http://ktci.education
- **TASHRA (The Alternative Sexualities Health Research Alliance):** www.tashra.org

Consensual nonmonogamy relationship structures are also common within queer communities, but not exclusively so.[10] Consensually nonmonogamous relationships encompass a wide variety of relationship structures and/or identities that have in common the foundation of open communication and agreement between all people involved about the nonmonogamous nature of the relationships.[11] *Polyamorous* is another term that describes identity and types of relationships, and refers to an approach to relationships that are open to forming loving relationships with multiple partners. People may generally describe their partnerships as "open relationships," which refers to maintaining close emotional intimacy or connections within a primary dyad but the partners may also pursue additional casual romantic or sexual partners either together or separately.[12] In general, consensual nonmonogamy is an umbrella term to describe relationship structures that operate outside of traditional norms of monogamy or relationship exclusivity between only two people.[10]

FURTHER INFORMATION ON CONSENSUAL NONMONOGAMY/POLYAMORY

- *The Polyamorists Next Door: Inside Multiple-Partner Relationships and Families* by Dr. Elizabeth Sheff
- **American Psychological Association Consensual Nonmonogamy Task Force:** www.apadivisions.org/division-44/publications/newsletters/division/2017/06/non-monogamy
- **Consensual Nonmonogamy Inclusive Practices Tool:** www.drheathschechinger.com/blog/cnm-inclusive-practices-tool

QUEER AS SOCIOPOLITICAL AFFILIATION

The origins of queer theory, which has historically recognized both power structures as well as sexual variance, are sometimes credited to the ideas of French philosopher Michel Foucault.[13] Foucault postulated that sexuality was not determined by genetics or biology but rather was socially constructed. This construction often depended on cultural norms and history;[14] for example, in classically Greco-Roman MSM sexual relationships that were not deemed "gay" (or queer) per se.[9] Foucault believed that within sex there were inherent power dynamics even in the creation of desire by culture and institutions. This included historical examples of "same-sex" relationships, for example, as previously referenced regarding Greco-Roman MSM relationships, which were considered normal between ambitious younger men and more powerful older ones. He also spoke of the need to claim sexuality as an important part of our culture, and as normal within its many variations.[13] The understanding that power differentials shape individual construction of desire (and its relationship to sexual variance) is central to queer community original definitions.

Foucault writes about this, describing what he says is a need to speak publicly without regard for the acknowledgment of the purported illicit nature of some types of sexuality, or the condemnation for sexuality in its variance, even if the speaker represents, themself, sexual variance. This was in order to assert the regularity of sexual variances into civil society, so that it could also be administered to, as were other parts of the individual, for the good of all people.[13]

Many queer-identified people hold political beliefs that are a challenge to existing mainstream ideologies. These individuals and communities may identify as queer in order to build community with like-minded people who may not hold the same sexual attractions.[9] Within queer communities and individuals there can be a rejection of "normalcy" frameworks that mainstream LGB-identified people are more likely to choose. Individuals may see "queerness" as a choice for their identity because it is an umbrella identity that encompasses a spectrum of genders and sexualities. This can be an intentional way to create community with many different types of people who are LGBTQIA+. In multiple cities in the world, there are now "Queer Pride" parades versus LGBT or Gay Pride Parades, often intentional choices to encompass the multidimensional identities within the communities.[15]

PROVIDING CULTURALLY SAFE CARE FOR PEOPLE WHO IDENTIFY AS QUEER

The five tenets of cultural safety—*partnerships, personal ADLs, prevention of harm, patient centering,* and *purposeful self-reflection*—are central to creating safety for patients who identify as queer.[16]

For example, when *partnering* with a patient who is queer, the power of elucidating sexual identity should be left to the patient themselves, and that if patients choose to offer identity clarification, the provider should be welcoming. Ensure that the clinical environment is such that when and if patients choose to clarify sexual identity, clinical staff are welcoming. The provider must understand that the patient is a leader and a healthcare partner in their own sexual and other health and avoid dictating or proffering sexual identity terminology.[17]

When respecting a patient's *personal ADLs*, understand that, as a clinician, all of the information about oppression or exclusion that a patient may have faced within a clinical setting can color their interest in frankly disclosing about themselves. Providers should research on their own time any confusing or unfamiliar information that a queer patient reveals. Additionally, the provider should choose to ask only the necessary healthcare questions while allowing space for anything further the patient might wish to share.[16]

Preventing harm is crucial to queer patient care. Frequent check-ins and support for any lifestyle decisions (including underground economy jobs) are vital to creating safety. Additionally, when entering the exam room, providers should introduce themselves to individual patients, while displaying body language that shows openness. Using active listening skills shows active engagement with the patient and their healthcare. Queer-identified people need to know through a provider's body language and words that they will not be forced to compartmentalize, or hide aspects of their lives, in order to receive quality healthcare.

When providing *patient-centered* care, consider that, for example, the provider's imperative to do primary prevention (like PrEP or pregnancy prevention) may not be aligned with queer patient needs. Offering multiple resources and interventions without assuming patients will agree to use them is one strategy for patient-centered care, while avoiding penalizing patients because their decisions differ from the ones that have been recommended is another. Providers have no jurisdiction or control over queer patients' sexualities or gender and should not expect queer patients' activities or self-definitions to be meaningful in the clinical environment. Simply put, the patient has no responsibility to present their lives in a way that is clinically clear or legible to the provider. It is only imperative that the provider's recommendations make reasonable sense (or are legible) to the patient.[18]

When providers feel emotional or have an unconscious reaction upon hearing certain information that a queer patient has provided (for example, if someone discloses about having sex with multiple partners in a consensually nonmonogamous relationship structure called a polycule), the provider's reaction is often due to a lack of *purposeful self-reflection*.[19] A provider may only be familiar with certain aspects of queerness from reading this chapter, and many things may come up in the clinical visit that are new and surprising. Self-reflection must be practiced regularly, and one strategy is to take note of what was surprising or new (such as the term *polycule*) as an indication that the provider should do further research on their own time using some of the resources provided in this book and elsewhere, so as to maintain focus during the clinical visit on providing appropriate care for the patient.

EMBRACING AMBIGUITY

In order to validate and fully recognize queer patients' lives and identities, providers must also embrace ambiguity and shifts within communities and individuals—and seek only to quantify these shifts in ways that are congruous to patient care. Scientific research is sparse regarding queer identity, with much of it focused on health outcomes. In a 2018 study, participants recognized the impacts of paternalism in healthcare and lack of understanding of marginalized population disparities in provider competencies.[20] Closely related, significant disparities have also been shown between providers' attitudes and actual clinical practices. For example, almost 80% of healthcare providers purported comfort in the treatment of LGBTQIA+ patients while even recognizing that LGBTQIA+ populations have specialized health risks and needs (90.6%); however, over 70% of these providers also revealed not feeling well informed on the health needs or clinical management of LGBTQIA+ health needs, or on methods referring to patients with LGBTQ issues (78.7%).[21]

Even while taking the potential impact of racism out of the clinical environment, white queer patients also claim to not feel comfortable with healthcare providers, with 25% of LGBTQIA+-identified patients in a 2017 qualitative study reporting a negative attitude shift when providers find out their identities and a white cisgender lesbian reporting, "It's so uncomfortable to be talking to a doctor and then they treat you differently once they find out."[20] These participants recommended that competency development should be done alongside patients to more comprehensively ensure that gaps in provider knowledge are filled so that providers may develop the necessary skills to build collaboration with patients.[20]

APPROACHING SEXUAL HEALTH FOR QUEER PATIENTS

Approaching queer patients in a culturally safe manner actually mirrors good care for all patients and includes: lack of unnecessary curiosity, embracing patients' identities, and support of patient through knowledge of their *personal ADLs*. When asking questions that relate to patients' sexual health, consider the following clinical pathway:

1. Ask about activity before asking about sexual identity. You can start with:
    "When was the last time you were screened for STIs?"
    "Were there reasons or symptoms that prompted your screening for STIs in (month/year) OR every (interval)?"

    And perhaps:
    "Have you ever been treated for an STI?"
    "When was the last time you were treated for an STI?"

2. When asking about sexual activity, consider asking questions as introduction questions:
    "Are you physically intimate with any partners currently?"
    "Are you currently sleeping with anyone?"
    "Are you dating anyone at the moment?"

3. Next, or alternatively, if you feel that the patient is very comfortable discussing their sexuality, consider the following questions:
    "What kind of sex are you having?"
    "What body parts are you generally using for sexual activity?"

Pointed or closed-ended-questions that name identities, such as, "Are you a lesbian?" or "Are you gay?" do not actually help providers understand healthcare needs of the patient. Queer patients often fare best in sexual health situations when they are aware that their whole selves are welcome without overt pointed questioning about their sexualities or labels.[18] This means avoiding questions about sexual identity words or offering words that would label identity for someone else. Asking about sexual health and intimate and important relationships can prompt patients to reveal their preferred language around their own sexual identity, which should be greeted neutrally or positively.

CULTURAL SAFETY SUMMARY POINTS

As the landscape of LGBTQIA+ health continues to expand, clinicians must recognize the scarcity of LGBTQIA+-focused curricula available to clinicians in training.[22,23] This is despite the increased need for services for this community. By augmenting one's own knowledge base, individual providers will increase their levels of confidence in working with queer individuals. The hope is that this increased confidence will affect patient care in a positive way. The more clinicians embrace learning from queer patients about their own selves, the better care will be. This may mean researching local and national resources that are available in both formal and informal networks and providing appropriate recommendations to patients as indicated.

CONCLUSION

- Definitions and historical background of queerness are complex, variable, and nonstatic.
- Queer is an umbrella term applied to multidimensional sexual orientations, gender identities, gender expressions, and sexual behaviors.
- Some may reject the term *queer* due to its historically pejorative usage.

Case Study 6.1

Carson is a 48-year-old trans masculine nonbinary patient who comes in for STI screening as well as primary care. He states that he is excited to be coming to you because he heard that you are "queer-friendly" and can handle patients whose sexual activities are not normally cared for properly in many primary care settings.

What questions would you ask Carson?

How do you ensure that your care is supporting Carson's overall health including his sexuality?

REFERENCES

1. Drescher J. Queer diagnoses: parallels and contrasts in the history of homosexuality, gender variance, and the diagnostic and statistical manual. *Arch Sex Behav.* 2010;39(2):427–460. doi:10.1007/s10508-009-9531-5

2. Chmielewski JF, Belmonte KM, Fine M, et al. Intersectional inquiries with LGBTQ and gender nonconforming youth of color: participatory research on discipline disparities at the race/sexuality/gender nexus. In: Skiba RJ, Mediratta K, Rausch MK, eds. *Inequality in School Discipline: Research and Practice to Reduce Disparities.* Palgrave Macmillan; 2016:171–188. doi:10.1057/978-1-137-51257-4_10

3. Turner GW, Pelts M, Thompson M. Between the academy and queerness: microaggressions in social work education. *Affilia.* 2018;33(1):98–111. doi:10.1177/0886109917729664

4. Human Rights Campaign. Glossary of terms. 2018. https://www.hrc.org/resources/glossary-of-terms

5. Everyday Feminism. 3 differences between the terms "gay" and "queer"—and why it matters. Published March 1, 2016. https://everydayfeminism.com/2016/03/difference-between-gay-queer

6. Stief M. The sexual orientation and gender presentation of Hijra, Kothi, and Panthi in Mumbai, India. *Arch Sex Behav.* 2017;46(1):73–85. doi:10.1007/s10508-016-0886-0

7. Scott L. South Africa needs to find a new way to talk about being gay. *The Guardian.* Published January 27, 2015. https://www.theguardian.com/world/2015/jan/27/-sp-south-africa-gay-lesbian-bisexual-lgbti-language-isixhosa

8. Waldura JF, Arora I, Randall AM, et al. Fifty shades of stigma: exploring the health care experiences of kink-oriented patients. *J Sex Med.* 2016;13(12):1918–1929. doi:10.1016/j.jsxm.2016.09.019

9. McGuire L. Adding 'K' to LGBTQIA: is kink inherently queer? *Spectrum South—Voice Queer South.* February 2019. https://www.spectrumsouth.com/queer-kink

10. Levine EC, Herbenick D, Martinez O, et al. Open relationships, nonconsensual nonmonogamy, and monogamy among U.S. adults: findings from the 2012 National Survey of Sexual Health and Behavior. *Arch Sex Behav.* 2018;47(5):1439–1450. doi:10.1007/s10508-018-1178-7

11. American Psychology Association. Toward inclusive science and practice. 2017. https://www.apadivisions.org/division-44/publications/newsletters/division/2017/06/non-monogamy

12. Schippers M. *Beyond Monogamy: Polyamory and the Future of Polyqueer Sexualities.* New York University Press; 2016.

13. Foucault M. *The History of Sexuality.* 1st American ed. Pantheon Books; 1978.

14. Foucault M. *The History of Sexuality.* Vol 1. Pantheon Books; 1926.

15. Riemer M, Brown L. *We Are Everywhere: Protest, Power, and Pride in the History of Queer Liberation.* Potter/Ten Speed/Harmony/Rodale; 2019.

16. Kellett P, Fitton C. Supporting transvisibility and gender diversity in nursing practice and education: embracing cultural safety. *Nurs Inq.* 2017;24(1):e12146. doi:10.1111/nin.12146

17. Wesp LM, Scheer V, Ruiz A, et al. An emancipatory approach to cultural competency: the application of critical race, postcolonial, and intersectionality theories. *Adv Nurs Sci.* 2018;41(4):316–326. doi:10.1097/ANS.0000000000000230

18. Baker K, Beagan B. Making assumptions, making space: an anthropological critique of cultural competency and its relevance to queer patients: making assumptions, making space. *Med Anthropol Q.* 2014;28(4):578–598. doi:10.1111/maq.12129

19. Sheff E, Wolf T. *Stories From the Polycule: Real Life in Polyamorous Families*. Thorntree Press LLC; 2015.

20. Alpert AB, CichoskiKelly EM, Fox AD. What lesbian, gay, bisexual, transgender, queer, and intersex patients say doctors should know and do: a qualitative study. *J Homosex*. 2017;64(10):1368–1389. doi:10.1080/00918369.2017.1321376

21. Nowaskie DZ, Sowinski JS. Primary care providers' attitudes, practices, and knowledge in treating LGBTQ communities. *J Homosex*. 2019;66(13):1927–1947. doi:10.1080/00918369 .2018.1519304

22. White W, Brenman S, Paradis E, et al. Lesbian, gay, bisexual, and transgender patient care: medical students' preparedness and comfort. *Teach Learn Med*. 2015;27(3):254–263. doi: 10.1080/10401334.2015.1044656

23. Lim FA, Brown DV, Justin Kim SM. Addressing health care disparities in the lesbian, gay, bisexual, and transgender population. *Am J Nurs*. 2014;114(6):24–34. doi:10.1097/01 .NAJ.0000450423.89759.36

7

Asexual Patient Care

Ronica Mukerjee and Poonam Daryani

LEARNING OBJECTIVES

By the end of this chapter, the reader will be able to:

- Understand some issues that asexual patients experience in clinical environments.
- Describe some recommendations in caring for asexual patients.
- List some ways to support patients who identify as asexual.

INTRODUCTION

A multidimensional, culturally competent and affirmative approach that takes into account self-identification, attraction, and behavior is recommended when offering clinical care to asexual patients.[1,2] Clinicians must avoid pathologizing the lack of sexual activity or sexual interest that asexual patients may have and instead see the sexual identity/identities that asexual patients may have as various and intersecting, including with other LGBTQIA+ identities. In fact, culturally safe care for asexual patients is often a good recipe for culturally safe care for many other types of patients.

While asexuality is generally defined as a sexual orientation describing someone who does not experience sexual attraction,[3] this definition is actively debated within the literature and asexual communities: There have been arguments for definitions based on self-identification (rather than attraction)[3]; re-framings of asexuality as a radical disruption of norms privileging sexuality (rather than as a lack of something)[4–6]; and suggestions that asexuality be thought of as a "meta-category, just like *sexual*" that encompasses a range of desire, attraction and behavior-related constructs (rather than as a single sexual orientation).[3,7] To the latter point that asexuality might be better understood as a "meta-category" or umbrella term, Table 7.1 sheds light on the enormous diversity of asexual spectrum identities, including a plurality of

(a) romantic orientations and various types and degrees of attractions and desires. For clinicians, this heterogeneity means that different patients will differently understand, describe, and experience their asexuality.

It is also important to note that the academic and asexual community generally do not support behavior-based definitions of asexuality (i.e., a lack of participation in sexual behavior).[3] It is well established that asexuals and non-asexuals alike may engage in solitary and partnered sexual activity for complex and diverse motives other than sexual attraction, including but not limited to: curiosity; desire, obligation, pressure, or coercion to please a partner; pressure to conform to social expectations of sexuality; relaxation and tension release; involvement in the sex trade sector; and so on.[1,6,8,9]

THE PATHOLOGIZATION OF ASEXUALITY

Asexuality as a pathology and site of medical and psychiatric intervention has its roots in the sexual sciences, including sexology and psychiatric science, which are premised on the belief that sexuality is biologically innate and universal to all human beings.[4] This essentializing ideology, often referred to as "sexual normativity," "compulsory sexuality," or "sexusociety," assumes all people are sexual unless otherwise specified and privileges sexuality as ideal and superior.[3,5] The coding of sexuality— and particularly heterosexuality—as normal (i.e., "healthy"), ubiquitous, and imperative turns differences in sexuality into abnormalities and provides the rationale for the establishment of "sexual dysfunctions" as a category within psychiatric science.

The 1980 Third Edition of the American Psychiatric Association's *Diagnostic and Statistical Manual of Mental Disorders* (*DSM-III*®) was the first to include the diagnostic category of "Inhibited Sexual Desire," subsequently renamed in the *DSM-IV* "Hypoactive Sexual Desire Disorder" (HSDD), a psychiatric diagnosis characterized by a deficiency or absence of sexual fantasies and desire for sexual activity, causing marked distress or interpersonal difficulty.[4,10]

Notably, the *DSM-5* released in 2013 separated the criteria for HSDD into different disorders for females and males: Female Sexual Interest Desire/Arousal Disorder (FSAID) and Male Hypoactive Sexual Desire Disorder (MHSDD). This restructuring reportedly was done with the intention of acknowledging that sexual desire might be experienced differently by men and women (for instance, there is recognition that women's low sexual desire may be the product of intimate partner violence, which would preclude diagnosis of FSAID).[11] However, the binary restructuring erases the existence of many intersex, gender nonconforming, genderfluid, agender, and other gender variant peoples and may create conditions for asexual women who come to asexuality later in life or after periods of sexuality to be disproportionately pathologized.[7]

Clinicians should avoid presuming pathology in patients who describe themselves as experiencing little or no sexual attraction, whether or not they identify as asexual. The discourse around how clinicians should distinguish between HSDD and asexuality has largely centered on the "marked distress" criteria in the diagnosis. However, as many have noted, this parameter does not account for how social experiences and power inequities along many intersecting axes—including the stigma and marginalization people may experience for being asexual—can contribute significantly to feelings of distress and impact functioning.[2,11]

One study, for instance, found that heterosexual people are more willing to discriminate against and dehumanize asexual people than other sexual minority groups: Heterosexual participants characterized asexual people as "machine-like" (cold and emotionless) and "animal-like" (less sophisticated), suggesting a belief that sexuality is a key component of humanness.[12] In another study, two-thirds of asexually-identified interviewees reported occasionally feeling isolated or alienated from others or from society due to the stigmatization and invisibility of non-sexual identities in a sexusociety.[6] It is worth mentioning that these experiences of negation are not absent in feminist, queer, and LGBT+ spaces, where asexual people are at times treated as sexually repressed and unliberated, and, in some cases, as threats to the sex-positive movement.[13] Moreover, the distress and interpersonal difficulty experienced by an asexual person may be mediated by other social relations of power, such as gender, race, class, and disability. Distress is not felt in a vacuum: The fact that there are diverse and varied sources of distress, particularly in the context of a society that devalues and can be outright hostile to non-sexualities, is the first fault line in the HSDD criteria.

The second major fault line is that relying on "distress" to separate asexuality from sexual desire disorders creates a dichotomy between the "real" asexual who is happy, well-adjusted, and healthy (not dealing with mental health issues) versus a pathological non-sexual who warrants medical intervention and corrective treatment.[11] In the latter case of someone who *is* distressed about their low sexual desire, arguments have been made that their needs may not be best served by a diagnosis of HSDD. In the case of a patient experiencing significant distress who has not yet encountered asexuality, a provider may offer relevant information and resources on asexuality as a natural sexual variation and a potentially fulfilling identity, before concluding a diagnosis of HSDD.[3] Additionally, most people diagnosed with HSDD are heterosexual women experiencing an unwanted decrease in sexual desire while in romantic relationships with men who desire more sex from them: In this context, it is important to name the strong social controls prescribing and policing female (hetero)sexuality.[11] Individuals who want medical or mental health attention for low or no sexual desire should have the agency and ability to seek a diagnosis and intervention.[10] In the same vein, if after thoughtful evaluation, a provider and patient agree that a diagnosis of HSDD is appropriate and/or that increasing levels of sexual desire is the therapeutic goal, this should be paired with actions that interrogate and transform norms making sexual desire compulsory. As researcher Chasin has stated, asexual people may not want sex, just like anyone else. If this can be OK—asexual people not desiring sexual contact—then maybe this can be acceptable for any human, with no mandate that sexual activity is always part and parcel of normalcy or intimacy or obligatory to prove emotional closeness. Chasin writes that if no person is made to feel that their lack of sexual desire is pathological, then any person, asexual or not, may feel less concerned with changing their levels of desire for sex.[11]

The pathologization of asexuality by healthcare providers does not always happen directly via a *DSM* diagnosis. For instance, questioning someone's asexual identity as an unhealthy attitude toward sex, minimizing it as sexual immaturity (i.e., believing someone will enjoy sex once they try it), or assuming that asexuality is the product of adverse childhood experiences or sexual trauma also function as modes of pathologization.[6]

For healthcare providers, disassociating asexuality from a presumptive pathology means abandoning preconceived notions of (a)sexuality. Providers can instead appreciate that coming to an identity is a deeply personal social-psychological process influenced by one's unique structural, political, economic, and cultural context.[14] Recognizing that many paths can lead to an asexual identity and that identities can shift over time challenges the notion that (a)sexuality is biologically determined, innate, and unchanging. This may seem counterintuitive, as people with marginalized sexualities often assert essentializing claims (e.g., "I was born this way" or "asexuality is an intrinsic part of who we are"),[15] particularly when trying to establish legitimacy, and may genuinely feel that their (a)sexuality is a fixed and natural part of their identity. Although essentialism is resonant with many minoritized people and useful when differentiating asexuality from a pathology (e.g., HSDD) or other non-sexualities (e.g., celibacy), it perpetuates the belief that if asexuality is chosen or acquired (instead of inborn and lifelong), then it can and should be "corrected." Biological essentialism thereby upholds sexuality as the ideal outcome, rather than creating space for asexuality to be a valid and fulfilling way of being-in-the-world, without justification.[11]

Additionally, understanding (a)sexuality to be both individually-negotiated and socially-constructed enables providers to care for their patients more fully and competently.[6,14] As an example, the role of trauma in identity formation can be contentious for some asexual people given historical tendencies to *assume* asexuality is the undesirable and abnormal product of childhood and/or sexual trauma. However, providers who understand that a tangle of human experiences and power relations shapes one's social functioning and sense of self can explore the influence trauma may have had on an asexual patient without using it to delegitimize or pathologize their identity.[16] As one gender nonconforming South Asian writer expressed, in the context of racialized violence against people of color living under white supremacy in the United States, it is near impossible for them to extricate their asexuality from the historical and ongoing trauma of Asian men being socially de-emasculated and de-sexualized, not seen as worthy objects or subjects of desire.[17] For them, asexuality is not an identity they feel they can freely and proudly claim, but instead one lodged in storied histories of racialized violence. In this case, the root of the problem is deeply societal—not an individual pathology to be cured. Using a structurally competent and trauma-informed lens, providers can validate and support a patient in navigating *both* their asexual identity and the various forms of trauma they may have experienced and been impacted by.

ASEXUAL (ACE) IDENTITY AND RELATIONSHIPS

People who identify as asexual or as having one of the identities that fall into the spectrum of asexuality (Table 7.1) have multiple other identities and orientations.

TABLE 7.1 Examples of Asexual Identity Terms	
SOME ASEXUAL TERMS PATIENTS MAY USE	**WORKING DEFINITION**
Aromantic	Individuals who experience little or no romantic attraction
Asexual	Individuals who, in the spectrum of asexuality, may not experience sexual attraction
Akoisexual/Akoiromantic	Individuals who stop experiencing sexual or romantic attraction when those feelings are reciprocated
Aceflux/Aroflux	Individuals who have sexual and romantic orientations that may vary within the spectrum of asexual/sexual, and aromantic/romantic
Demisexual	Individuals who experience sexual attraction only in the context of having an emotional connection or longer-term relationship with someone, often in romantic relationships
Grey-A/Grey asexual	Possibly overlapping types: Some Grey-A individuals <ul><li>Do not regularly experience sexual attraction but can sometimes</li><li>Experience sexual attraction but do not have sexual desire</li><li>Experience attraction and desire but do not regularly act on them</li><li>Enjoy sexual activity but in limited circumstances</li></ul>
Reciprosexual/Recipromantic	Individuals do not experience sexual/romantic feelings unless another individual is sexually attracted to or romantically interested in them

Source: Data from Carrigan M. There's more to life than sex? Difference and commonality within the asexual community. *Sexualities*. 2011;14(4):462–478. doi:10.1177/1363460711406462; Gupta K. "And now I'm just different, but there's nothing actually wrong with me": asexual marginalization and resistance. *J Homosex*. 2017;64(8):991–1013. doi:10.1080/00918369.2016.1236590; Pasquier M. Explore the spectrum: guide to finding your Ace community. amp. 2018. https://www.glaad.org/amp/ace-guide-finding-your-community

Importantly, identifying as asexual does not define the other attractions one may experience. In fact, asexuals vary in (a) the types of attraction and desire they experience (e.g., sexual, romantic, sensual, intellectual, etc.), (b) the levels of attraction and desire they experience along a fluid continuum (e.g., demisexual, grey-A), and (c) the genders toward which they experience attraction and desire.[3]

To illustrate some of the diversity: Asexual people may identify as queer, lesbian, bi, straight, or any combination of these and other orientation and identity categories. Being asexual does not foreclose desire for sensuality, intimacy, and pleasure. Many asexuals desire and engage in meaningful and emotionally-connected relationships with others, including romantic relationships (though aromantic asexuals are also an important part of the community and should not be overlooked). Some may experience sexual attraction, but have no desire to act on that attraction. Others may experience sexual desire, but feel no sexual attraction toward anyone or anything. Some asexuals may desire physical affection and intimacy, including acts sexualized in Western culture, such as kissing or cuddling, which they experience as non-sexual (scholars have noted the radicalness of this de-sexualization in disrupting definitions of sex and exposing its subjectivity).[6,14] While some asexuals have positive attitudes toward sex and simply do not want to participate in it themselves, others find it deeply repulsive and distressing.[18]

Though more information on demographics is needed, there are indications of gender differences in the prevalence of asexuality: Some studies have found a greater proportion of women than men who self-identify as asexual (though this may reflect some study volunteer bias), as well as significant gender diversity in terms of people who are trans-identified or who do not conform with conventional binary categories of gender and biological sex (i.e., they identify as intersex, genderqueer, agender, genderfluid, etc.).[3,8] By being aware of the multiplicity of identities and attitudes within the asexual population, providers can cultivate a safe space and affirming practice for patients to bring their "whole selves" into a clinical setting.[2]

INTERSECTIONALITY, DISABILITY, AND ASEXUALITY

Because identities are multi-layered and intersectional, asexuality should always be considered alongside intersecting axes of oppression and privilege, including race, gender, class, and disability. In particular, as Eunjung Kim writes, "because normative sexual desire and personhood have been historically centered around heterosexuality, maleness, whiteness and able-bodiedness, an examination of pathologized constructions of asexuality reveals their gendered, raced, and embodied dimensions as well as heterosexual assumptions."[19]

In the context of asexuality, there is a long and fraught history of de-sexualization of people whose bodies fall outside of normative bounds: People who are disabled, elderly, intersex, children, lesbian, transgender, or racialized as "other" have, in different and overlapping moments, been *denied* sexuality and have had asexuality imposed or assumed.[19] It is also important to note that other groups have been subjected to the opposite construction (hypersexualization), in which a presumed "excess" of sexuality has been pathologized and even criminalized (for instance, people who sell or trade sex historically have been branded as vectors of disease and made targets of state control via the criminal law and other penal institutions). The racialized trope of Black women as asexual and docile mammy figures, which was fabricated in order to soothe white anxieties of Blackness in white homes and near white children, can be juxtaposed with the hypersexualization of Black women as out-of-control jezebels, which provided a rationale for racist violence and discipline.[20] In these scenarios and in many others, sexual normativity is mobilized to define the boundaries of humanity and to distribute benefits to those within bounds and to subordinate those outside. While there are important differences between self-proclaimed asexual movements and identities and the ascribed de-sexualization of people as a mechanism of oppression, health-care providers must be aware of how sexual normativity has impacted differently situated groups.

Honing in on asexuality and disability, the characterization of asexuality as a disorder and of disabled people as asexual has led to mutual negation, in which both groups have at times excluded or repudiated the other in efforts to depathologize their respective identities.[19,21] Whereas disability groups have sought recognition via claims of sexual normalcy, asexual groups have sought recognition via claims of bodily normalcy and healthiness (i.e., emphasizing that they do not have physical or cognitive disabilities).[19,21]

While patients with disabilities may indeed identify as asexual, providers should not assume that lack of appropriate technology or aids to have sex in satisfying ways means that patients are not considering or desirous of sexual activity. To the contrary, providers should be attentive and responsive to the various institutional, structural, and cultural barriers disabled patients may face in sexual expression.[21] Moreover, for asexual-identified disabled patients, providers should be aware of their risk of double erasure and should provide appropriate healthcare that is sensitive to both identities.[19,22]

While there are some data that suggest increased prevalence of asexuality among autistic people, scholars have also noted that this may be because people on the autis-tic spectrum in general display greater diversity of sexuality and/or sexual orientation than the non-autistic population (i.e., less heterosexuality and more of everything else), meaning that the increased prevalence may not be due to any specific or causal relationship between asexuality and autism.[7]

BEST PRACTICES FOR PROVIDING CULTURALLY SAFE CARE FOR PEOPLE WHO IDENTIFY AS ASEXUAL

Primary care providers have a central and active role to play in providing inclu-sive, affirming, and competent patient care for asexual patients. Given the histo-ries of pathologization of asexuality by medical institutions, many asexual patients expect practitioner bias: Even when they conceive of their asexuality as a healthy part of their identity, they may anticipate being dismissed or pathologized by pro-viders, and this distrust can at times be a deterrent to seeking care.[2] In one study with asexually-identified individuals, half of the interviewees reported experiences of pathologization by a medical provider.[6] We review some recommendations for how primary care providers working with patients experiencing low or no sexual at-traction (whether or not they identify as on the asexual spectrum) can prioritize the goals of the patient, provide safe and affirming care, and counteract pathologization or stigmatization.[2,10]

1. Providers should avoid assigning identities to patients based on their sexual behavior and instead privilege the patient's agency by allowing them to self-identify and describe themselves.
2. Providers should assess whether asexual patients are engaging in sexual activity and follow protocols for providing affirming sexual healthcare, including STI screening based on orifices and body parts used. Remember that having an active sex life does not alter the asexual identity that the patient may have.
3. Providers can actively signal to patients that they are accepting and affirming of asexual identities and more generally the full spectrum of sexual variation, such as by using gender-neutral language when asking about sexual history and explicitly including "asexuality" as an option on demographic intake forms[2] or allowing for open-ended responses so that patients can self-identify using the language they prefer. The enormous diversity of identities within the (a)sexual umbrella are difficult to capture in mutually exclusive sexual orientation categories.[3] Moreover, understandings of terms will vary across patients, as illustrated by the fact that there is no consistently and uniformly accepted definition of asexuality.[3] Providers can also have informational materials on asexuality visible and available for patients. For instance, the Asexual Visibility and Education Network (AVEN) is the largest community for asexual people and allies, offering online information, discussion boards, and resources as well as offline community building and advocacy opportunities.
4. When presented with a patient (whether or not they identify as asexual) with significant distress related to their level of sexual attraction or desire, providers should carefully evaluate the sources of distress through a trauma-informed and intersectional lens that considers the patient's socio-cultural context and their identities across lines of race, gender, disability, and class. The provider should consider the expectations, pressures, and stigmatization the patient may be facing, which may stem from a partner with whom they are in a relationship or, more broadly, from a sexual society that naturalizes and universalizes sexuality. Providers have a responsibility to inform patients of their full range of options, including about HSDD and available treatment options as well as about asexuality and the asexual community, and to grant them the agency to determine for themselves if either label is appropriate.[10] If a patient is seeking treatment due to discrepancy in levels of sexual desire with a partner, the couple should be referred to relationship therapy with the goal of improving communication and developing agreements that appease both partners, rather than the person with lower sexual interest being taught sexual skills or receiving pharmacological and/or hormonal treatment.[10,23]

5. Providers should focus on addressing the patient's presenting health issues without placing undue attention on their asexual identity if not clinically relevant.
6. Providers should be engaged in an ongoing process of critical self-reflection that challenges their own biases and increases their knowledge of human sexual variation and skills on providing inclusive, affirming, and structurally competent care to all patients.

CULTURAL SAFETY SUMMARY POINTS

- *Partnering* with patients involves using gender-neutral language when asking about sexual history and explicitly including "asexuality" as an option on demographic intake forms, having informational materials on asexuality visible and available for patients, and connecting with communities for asexual people to explore advocacy opportunities.
- *Prevention of harm* occurs through a trauma-informed and intersectional lens that considers expectations, pressures, and stigmatization the patient may be facing within personal relationships or broader societal expectations.
- Providers should engage in *purposeful self-reflection* that challenges any implicit biases about human sexual variation.

CONCLUSION

- Asexuality is an umbrella term that encompasses various and varied gender identities, orientations, levels of desire, forms of attraction, and ranges of (a)sexual expression.
- Preliminary demographic information indicates a significant amount of gender diversity within Ace identity.
- Providers can increase competency of care by being informed about the multiplicity of identities and attitudes within Ace population.
- Clinicians must avoid pathologizing asexuality and instead have it be understood as an identity.
- Asexual identity may be varied and intersecting and may be part of LGBTQIA+ identity.
- Self-identification and re-framing of asexuality as a radical disruption of norms provides an alternate and non-pathologizing definition of this identity.
- Asexuality may be conceptualized as a "meta-category" that includes a spectrum of non-homogeneous identities.
- Academia and the asexual community alike do not support behavior-based definitions of asexuality.
- An asexual individual may or may not participate in sexual behavior.

Case Study 7.1

Jay is a 28-year-old non-binary AFAB (assigned female at birth) person who identifies as asexual and presents to your office for a primary care visit including sexual health screening. Jay uses they/them pronouns and speaks to you about hiding their identity from their partner, during their work as a sex worker, and also with their family who expect Jay to one day have children and be a good wife. How would you approach this patient with multiple identities in giving them the primary care they should receive?

While acknowledging Jay's multiple identities, consider what health issues may be occurring for Jay as a result of their personal identities, relationship needs, and workplace exposures. Of course, Jay will have primary care needs that are typical for all patients of their age and physiology; for example, screening bloodwork and other needed preventive care including HPV testing as needed. As a clinician, you will also want to address the health of their relationship with their partner: for example, are they safe or in a consensual relationship? This will likely not be just a first encounter conversation but a conversation to broach in order to create room for the patient to have this conversation in a safe, non-personal setting. Also, Jay's STI prevention and screening needs must be addressed with appropriate orifice screening as well as prevention as needed. This must be done in a way that acknowledges that these interventions for an Ace person might be dysphoric to their innate identity but are protective of the body that Jay is using for work and possibly to maintain a relationship. Cultural/family pressures that Jay is experiencing must also be explored but this may happen more effectively over time.

REFERENCES

1. Van Houdenhove E, Gijs L, T'Sjoen G, et al. Stories about asexuality: a qualitative study on asexual women. *J Sex Marital Ther.* 2015;41(3):262–281. doi:10.1080/00926 23X.2014.889053
2. Foster AB, Scherrer KS. Asexual-identified clients in clinical settings: implications for culturally competent practice. *Psychol Sex Orientat Gend Divers.* 2014;1(4):422–430. doi:10.1037/sgd0000058
3. Chasin CD. Theoretical issues in the study of asexuality. *Arch Sex Behav.* 2011;40(4):713–723. doi:10.1007/s10508-011-9757-x
4. Flore J. Mismeasures of asexual desires. In: Cerankowski KJ, Milks M, eds. *Asexualities: Feminist and Queer Perspectives.* Routledge; 2014:31–48.
5. Przybylo E. Crisis and safety: the asexual in sexusociety. *Sexualities.* 2011;14(4):444–461. doi:10.1177/1363460711406461
6. Gupta K. "And now I'm just different, but there's nothing actually wrong with me": asexual marginalization and resistance. *J Homosex.* 2017;64(8):991–1013. doi:10.1080/00918369.2016.1236590

7. Chasin CD. Considering asexuality as a sexual orientation and implications for acquired female sexual arousal/interest disorder. *Arch Sex Behav.* 2017;46(3):631–635. doi:10.1007/s10508-016-0893-1

8. Brotto LA, Knudson G, Inskip J, et al. Asexuality: a mixed-methods approach. *Arch Sex Behav.* 2010;39(3):599–618. doi:10.1007/s10508-008-9434-x

9. Prause N, Graham CA. Asexuality: classification and characterization. *Arch Sex Behav.* 2007;36(3):341–356. doi:10.1007/s10508-006-9142-3

10. Gupta K. What does asexuality teach us about sexual disinterest? Recommendations for health professionals based on a qualitative study with asexually identified people. *J Sex Marital Ther.* 2017;43(1):1–14. doi:10.1080/0092623X.2015.1113593

11. Chasin CD. Reconsidering asexuality and its radical potential. *Feminist Stud.* 2013;39(2):405–426. https://www.jstor.org/stable/23719054

12. MacInnis CC, Hodson G. Intergroup bias toward "Group X": evidence of prejudice, dehumanization, avoidance, and discrimination against asexuals. *Group Process Intergroup Relat.* 2012;15(6):725–743. doi:10.1177/1368430212442419

13. Milks M. Stunted growth: asexual politics and the rhetoric of sexual liberation. In: Cerankowski KJ, Milks M, eds. *Asexualities: Feminist and Queer Perspectives.* Routledge; 2014:114–132.

14. Scherrer KS. Coming to an asexual identity: negotiating identity, negotiating desire. *Sexualities.* 2008;11(5):621–641. doi:10.1177/1363460708094269

15. The Asexual Visibility and Education Network. Overview. Accessed May 23, 2019. https://www.asexuality.org/?q=overview.html

16. Kurowicka A. Asexual affects: what abjection, anxiety and shame have to do with asexuality. Accessed May 27, 2019. https://www.academia.edu/30702756/Asexual_Affects_What_Abjection_Anxiety_and_Shame_Have_to_Do_with_Asexuality

17. Vaid-Menon A. What's r(ace) got to do with it?: white privilege & (a)sexuality. Media Diversified. Published May 2014. https://mediadiversified.org/2014/05/03/whats-race-got-to-do-with-it-white-privilege-asexuality

18. Carrigan M. There's more to life than sex? Difference and commonality within the asexual community. *Sexualities.* 2011;14(4):462–478. doi:10.1177/1363460711406462

19. Kim E. Asexualities and disabilities in constructing sexual normalcy. In: Cerankowski KJ, Milks M, eds. *Asexualities: Feminist and Queer Perspectives.* Routledge; 2014:263–296.

20. Owen IH. On the racialization of asexuality. In: Cerankowski KJ, Milks M, eds. *Asexualities: Feminist and Queer Perspectives.* Routledge; 2014:133–150.

21. Cuthbert K. You have to be normal to be abnormal: an empirically grounded exploration of the intersection of asexuality and disability. *Sociology.* 2017;51(2):241–257. doi:10.1177/0038038515587639

22. Kim E. Asexuality in disability narratives. *Sexualities.* 2011;14(4):479–493. doi:10.1177/1363460711406463

23. Brotto LA, Yule MA. Physiological and subjective sexual arousal in self-identified asexual women. *Arch Sex Behav.* 2011;40(4):699–712. doi:10.1007/s10508-010-9671-7

8

Intersex Patient Care

Ronica Mukerjee

LEARNING OBJECTIVES

By the end of this chapter, the reader will be able to:

- Understand challenges that intersex patients experience in clinical environments.
- Describe some components of the most recent consensus guidelines.
- List some unique pelvic implications for people who are intersex.

INTRODUCTION

The prospect of giving quality primary care to patients with intersex conditions can be daunting for primary care providers, who have rarely been educated properly about the needs of intersex patients.[1] This lack of training can lead to providers unintentionally creating fearful responses, leading to frustration for intersex patients and family members. These negative emotions can be a result of non-evidence-based conversations regarding patients' risk of serious diseases or by using inappropriate terminology when referring to patients' body parts, including genitalia.[1-3] These issues in care provision can also include provider lack of understanding around psychosocial, primary care, or fertility needs. Patients can, unfortunately, experience inadequate, biased, and culturally unsafe care as a result.[2] This chapter will explore the answers to some questions that providers may have, including when there may be requirements for interventions outside the primary care setting. This chapter is not meant to be comprehensive in understanding the medical care and management of the intersex patient, but rather to provide basic information to create a culturally safe setting.[4]

BASIC MEDICAL TERMINOLOGY

In order to offer *patient-centered* care, the correct terminology for an intersex individual regarding their personhood should be defined by the patients themselves.[5] At times, intersex individuals are referred to as having differences/disorders of sex development (DSDs) but this has fallen out of favor by many community members, many of whom prefer the term *intersex* as a self-descriptor.[6] Thus, for the purpose of consistency and meeting chapter objectives, these authors will use the term *intersex*. Additionally, there is also some controversy about what actually constitutes a true intersex diagnosis, with some experts believing that conditions such as polycystic ovarian syndrome (PCOS) are also intersex states. However, individuals with PCOS may or may not consider themselves to be intersex.[1-3]

Patients may refer to themselves by many terms, but some clues to relevant diagnoses used by patients include: "I am a person with Klinefelter's syndrome" or descriptions of their chromosomal differences such as "I have XXY chromosomes." Verbal cues are crucial in this environment as intersex patients have historically experienced a significant lack of cultural safety in clinical environments with a history of medical experimentation and nonconsensual medical practices and surgeries. This lack of cultural safety has often originated in childhood with nonconsensual examinations and procedures, which were not guided by understanding of *personal activities of daily living (ADLs)* or *prevention of harm*.[4] Many clinicians do not understand the daily needs (*personal ADLs*) of this patient population and how to provide care that is normal and healthy for intersex patients. Nor do providers understand that patients will make decisions regardless of clinician counseling and shaped by the patient's own interest in engaging in hormonal and surgical interventions. *Prevention of harm* in supporting these patients' journeys toward health includes frequent, as-desired check-ins, especially as unexpected body changes may be happening to intersex children during adolescence.

RECOMMENDED METHODS OF CARE

Two methods of care for intersex patients are outlined in Table 8.1, with the intersex-affirming model of care being what is currently recommended. Unfortunately, the medical experiences of intersex people have often been shaped by clinicians who practice the concealment-centered rearing model, originated at Johns Hopkins Hospital by psychologist John Money in the 1960s.[2] This model focused on hiding that an individual has intersex traits and focused on training patients toward gender binary choices. Money's models encouraged clinicians, parents, and children to see their intersex states as aberrations. This model pathologized their bodies, resulting in the recommendation for clinical interventions and surgeries.[7]

The intersex-affirming model of care is now the recommended practice (see Table 8.1). An affirming approach is where parents of intersex children and intersex patients themselves should not be given reasons to doubt that intersex people can be healthy without medical interventions. Nor should patients be advised that

	HOPKINS' CONCEALMENT MODEL OF CARE (NOT RECOMMENDED)	INTERSEX-AFFIRMING METHOD OF CARE (RECOMMENDED)
METHODS OF CARE		
Clinician understanding of intersex patient care	• Intersex children, adolescents, and adults need emergent interventions. • Intersex conditions are undesirable and parents cannot learn to care for intersex children.	• Intersex children, adolescents, and adults need support, understanding, and interdisciplinary interventions. • Intersex conditions are normal and very few conditions require surgical/hormonal interventions.
Clinician interaction with intersex child/adolescent and family	• Infants, toddlers, and adolescents receive life-altering surgeries that are not needed. • Parents are taught that their children have life-threatening medical conditions that require urgent and regular interventions. • Genitalia are altered to fit gender expectations of clinicians.	• Consensual decision-making with patient (even in childhood) and family. • Interdisciplinary teams including healthcare providers assist family coping. • Few situations require rushed decisions/ procedures/hormonal interventions. • Surgical decisions requiring genitalia alterations require considerable amounts of counseling and consent.

TABLE 8.1 Methods of Care for Intersex Patients

Source: Data from Frader J, Alderson P, Asch A, et al. Health care professionals and intersex conditions. *Arch Pediatr Adolesc Med.* 2004;158(5):426. doi:10.1001/archpedi.158.5.426; Intersex Society of North America. About. Accessed February 24, 2020. https://isna.org/about; Jenkins TM, Short SE. Negotiating intersex: a case for revising the theory of social diagnosis. *Soc Sci Med.* 2017;175:91–98. doi:10.1016/j.socscimed.2016.12.047; Kwok F. The experiences of intersex individuals. The Pitt Pulse. Accessed February 11, 2020. http://www.thepittpulse.org/the-experiences-of-intersex-individuals.

their bodies are abnormal and therefore in need of emergent interventions. Intersex patients are rarely in medical danger as a result of their intersex states. Instead of assuming that patients are in clinical danger and need immediate treatment, clinicians should carefully research clinical manifestations and needs of intersex patients before offering any advice and consult with consensus statements or multiple available peer-reviewed clinical guidelines as well as consultations with available specialized endocrinologists.

MORE INFORMATION ABOUT CARING FOR INTERSEX PATIENTS:

- Cools M, Robeva R, Hall J, et al. Caring for individuals with a difference of sex development (DSD): a consensus statement. *Nat Rev Endocrinol*. 2018;14(7):415–429. doi:10.1038/s41574-018-0010-8.
- Warne GL, Hewitt JK. The medical management of disorders of sex development. In: Hutson J, Warne G, Grover S, eds. *Disorders of Sex Development*. Springer International Publishing; 2011:159–172.

CLINICAL CARE FOR ADULTS

Safe clinical care for intersex adults is generally relatively uncomplicated, and this should be the baseline understanding in primary care settings. This chapter will focus on the care of people with the most common types of intersex states. The following chromosomal differences occur most commonly in intersex individuals: gonadal dysgenesis, hypogonadism, congenital adrenal hyperplasia, and complete and partial androgen insensitivity syndromes.[6]

There are several ways to classify intersex disorders. One way is to refer to the underlying difference (for example, sex chromosomal intersex states; 46, XY intersex states; and 46, XX intersex states).[6] See Figures 8.1, 8.2, and 8.3. Many intersex states fall under multiple types of categorization. Intersex states can also be categorized as gonadal dysgenesis disorders, which indicates that gonadal maturation is altered causing dysfunction and perhaps alteration of the external gonads ranging from under-virilization to over-virilization.[8,9]

Some laboratory and imaging diagnostics can assist in diagnosing intersex patients, when the family wishes for diagnosis. For example, soon after birth, karyotyping infants with ambiguous genitalia with X and Y genetic probes can help in understanding chromosomal configuration. Laboratory testing of testosterone, 17-hydroxyprogesterone, gonadotropins, anti-Müllerian hormone, and serum electrolytes (to rule out salt-wasting congenital adrenal hyperplasia) can be desirable and minimally invasive for infants. If indicated, noninvasive abdominal and pelvic ultrasounds should be the first diagnostic imaging test with understanding of their limitations. For example, ultrasound is effective in detecting gonads in the inguinal region and for understanding Müllerian anatomy. In order to localize the urogenital sinus and to understand the positioning of the urethra and vagina in this sinus, retrograde genitogram is usually needed.[10] There are also times when hormone stimulation tests as well as laparoscopic evaluation may be indicated, particularly to understand gonadal functioning or when nonpalpable testes are noted.[10]

SOME COMMON INTERSEX DIFFERENCES

Sex Chromosomal Intersex States

Turner Syndrome (45, X; a sex chromosomal intersex state): This is the most common cause of gonadal dysgenesis and affects between one in 2,000 and one in 2,500 live births (see Figure 8.1). With Turner syndrome, there is primary ovarian failure, structural abnormalities, or loss of one X chromosome in individuals who appear phenotypically female. With Turner syndrome, there is often short stature and a webbed neck. There are often cardiac abnormalities in these patients that require treatment, low thyroid stimulating hormone (TSH), and a higher incidence of diabetes mellitus. If menses and breast development are desired by patients, hormonal treatment is usually required. However, despite the historical underestimation of these patients' intellectual abilities in the past, generally there are no cognitive delays in these patients.[6,11]

Klinefelter Syndrome (47, XXY; a sex chromosomal intersex state): This affects one of every 500 to 2,000 male-identified neonates who have the karyotype 47, XXY (see Figure 8.1). Occasionally these individuals will have a small hypospadic phallus with minimal scrotal development and may have undescended testicles.[12] Controversially, some experts believe that these patients may have issues with reading and language acquisition, but pediatric-trained clinicians should definitely not inform parents that their child will not be able to read or communicate as this is not well confirmed as an ongoing process. Klinefelter syndrome is often diagnosed in adolescence when a patient presents with delayed, incomplete pubertal development and small testes; these patients often present as tall phenotypically male boys with some gynecomastia. These individuals may be predisposed to germ cell tumors, hypothyroidism, diabetes mellitus, varicose veins, and other immunological disorders.[6,11]

Noonan Syndrome (RAS-MPK pathway; a sex chromosomal intersex state): Noonan syndrome (see Figure 8.1) occurs in one out of 1,000 to one out of 2,500 live births (RAS-MPK pathway seen) with 50% of the differences occurring in the *PTPN11* gene and up to 15% more occurring in *SOS1* genes. Most individuals (90%) with Noonan syndrome have congenital heart defects. Many individuals with Noonan syndrome also have short stature, facial dysmorphism, hypogonadism, and increased risk of deafness. In patients typically assigned male at birth, small undescended testes are seen, whereas patients assigned female at birth may sometimes have delayed puberty.[6]

46, XX Intersex States

Gonadal Dysgenesis Syndromes (in 46, XX intersex individuals): Two common gonadal dysgenesis syndromes are ovotesticular DSDs and primary ovarian insufficiency (see Figure 8.2). Individuals with ovotesticular DSDs may have various manifestations of their state, including palpable testes or occasionally a combination ovotestis.[6,10] Some patients may have potential for fertility regardless of their phenotypic appearance and should be advised of this.

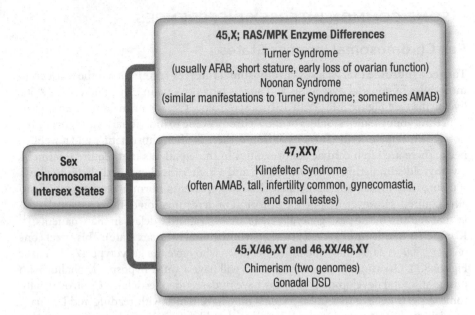

FIGURE 8.1 Some sex chromosomal differences.
AFAB, assigned female at birth; AMAB, assigned male at birth; DSD, difference of sex development.
Source: Data from Cools M, Robeva R, Hall J, et al. Caring for individuals with a difference of sex development (DSD): a consensus statement. *Nat Rev Endocrinol.* 2018;14(7):415–429. doi:10.1038/s41574-018-0010-8; Lee PA, Houk CP, Ahmed SF, et al. Consensus statement on management of intersex disorders. *Pediatrics.* 2006;118(2):e488–e500. doi:10.1542/peds.2006-0738.

Differences of Androgen Excess (a 46, XX intersex state): Aromatase deficiency, luteoma, and congenital or iatrogenic differences of androgen excess are common differences of androgen excess, which occurs in 8% of phenotypic female patients (see Figure 8.2). Androgen excess states are most common in phenotypically female patients; many body systems can be affected, although primarily the pilosebaceous systems with resulting hirsutism and reproductive systems are altered with resulting anovulatory infertility.[13] Aromatase deficiency is characterized by decreased levels of estrogen with elevated levels of testosterone. Phenotypic female individuals usually present with genitalia with both female and male characteristics with likely functional internal reproductive organs.[6] Luteoma in pregnancy can cause virilization of phenotypically female fetuses, which has typically been diagnosed as female pseudohermaphroditism.[14] Congenital and iatrogenic differences of androgen excess can include polycystic ovarian syndrome (PCOS), which can produce insulin insufficiency; this is particularly true in African Americans. Iatrogenic androgen excess also occurs with Cushing's syndrome, as a long-term result of medical treatment, specifically caused by a result of abnormally high cortisol and exogenous glucocorticoids.[13]

Unclassified Differences (46, XX intersex states): Mayer-Rokitansky-Kuster-Hauser syndromes types 1 and 2 (MRKH syndrome) (see Figure 8.2) occur most commonly in phenotypic females. This syndrome is associated with unremarkable external genitalia although the vagina and uterus can be underdeveloped or absent. When patients

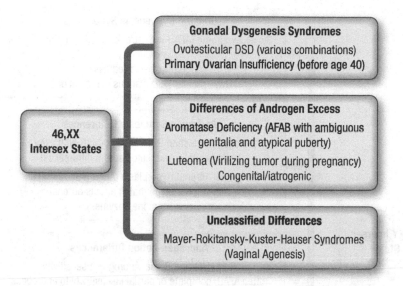

FIGURE 8.2 Some 46, XX differences.

AFAB, assigned female at birth; DSD, difference of sex development.

Source: Data from Cools M, Robeva R, Hall J, et al. Caring for individuals with a difference of sex development (DSD): a consensus statement. *Nat Rev Endocrinol.* 2018;14(7):415–429. doi:10.1038/s41574-018-0010-8; Lee PA, Houk CP, Ahmed SF, et al. Consensus statement on management of intersex disorders. *Pediatrics.* 2006;118(2):e488–e500. doi:10.1542/peds.2006-0738.

are affected, they typically do not menstruate; this is often the first sign of MRKH: primary amenorrhea, or absent menses by age 16. MRKH 2 usually involves renal and skeletal differences as well.[15]

Some 46, XY Intersex States

Gonadal Dysgenesis Syndromes (in 46, XY individuals): Swyer syndromes, anorchism, and ovotesticular DSDs are the most common gonadal dysgenesis syndromes (see Figure 8.3). Swyer syndrome in patients assigned female at birth is often associated with streak gonads and no noticeable puberty.[16] Anorchia can be associated with the absence or regression of one or more testes.[17] Ovotesticular DSDs of various combinations can have similar manifestations as 46, XX DSDs and have mixed or mosaic characteristics.[18]

Androgen Synthesis Syndrome Differences (in 46, XY intersex states): Androgen production differences and congenital adrenal hyperplasias (CAH) are the most common intersex states (see Figure 8.3). In androgen production differences, patients are generally assigned male at birth with external penises with testes and decreased sperm viability.[6] CAH affects adrenal gland function; the CAH states can including a salt-wasting form in which life-long corticosteroid treatment is necessary; ambiguous genitalia may be present in infants but also diagnosis can happen during atypical puberties.[19]

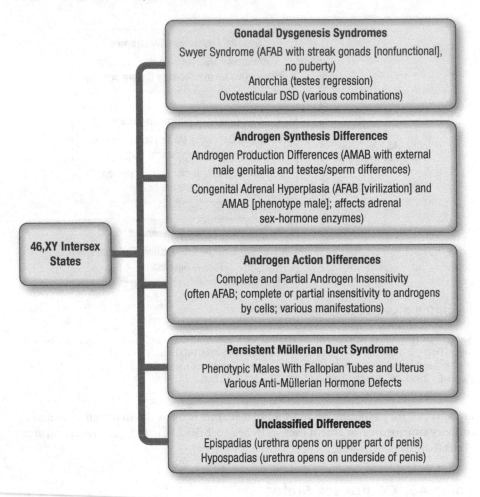

FIGURE 8.3 Some 46, XY differences.

AFAB, assigned female at birth; AMAB, assigned male at birth.

Source: Data from Cools M, Robeva R, Hall J, et al. Caring for individuals with a difference of sex development (DSD): a consensus statement. *Nat Rev Endocrinol.* 2018;14(7):415–429. doi:10.1038/s41574-018-0010-8; Lee PA, Houk CP, Ahmed SF, et al. Consensus statement on management of intersex disorders. *Pediatrics.* 2006;118(2):e488–e500. doi:10.1542/peds.2006-0738

Persistent Müllerian Duct Syndrome (in 46, XY intersex states): Persistent Müllerian duct syndrome (PMDS) generally affects individuals assigned male at birth and has been previously classified as a form of pseudohermaphroditism. Often these individuals have fallopian tubes and a uterus.[20]

Clinical Considerations

Gender Assignment: Inflexible gender assignments for intersex children should be discouraged. Although parents may experience alarm when they are not sure of correct sex assignment, clinicians should encourage parents to explore gender with their children in ways that acknowledge intersex children may not experience gender in the same manner that their non-intersex peers do. Mental health experts who are gender spectrum-affirming should be part of the gender needs of an intersex patient, whenever possible.[21]

Fertility Concerns: Likelihood of fertility in intersex patients depends on their intersex diagnosis. Generally, the fertility needs for intersex patients are not well understood. Unless a clinician is sure that a diagnosis precludes fertility, a patient should not be told they are infertile. Intersex people may, at times, find out both their fertility limitations or intersex condition when fertility attempts are unsuccessful. Both physiological and mental health interventions may be needed when this occurs. As with some other types of care for intersex patients, interdisciplinary care is often needed.

Androgen insensitivity syndrome (see Figure 8.3), a 46, XY intersex diagnosis, may be at the root of multiple types of infertility. There are experts who believe that AIS may be the primary source of infertility in most male-assigned patients. Patients with AIS and female-assignment typically do not develop internal female reproductive organs and are unable to conceive fetuses.[6]

That said, for many current adults with intersex diagnoses, fertility has not been decreased by their intersex diagnoses but rather from nonconsensual and other surgeries performed in childhood.

Cancer Risks: Some rare intersex diagnoses are associated with increased risk of germ cell cancers, most commonly in patients with gonadal dysgenesis.[6] For example, intraabdominal gonadal dysgenesis has a high associated risk of cancers with 15% to 35% of patients with this intersex diagnosis receiving a cancer diagnosis.[22] Nonscrotal partial androgen insensitivity syndrome (PAIS) has been associated with a 50% risk of malignancy. Gonadal biopsies may be warranted during adolescence.[6,22]

CULTURAL SAFETY SUMMARY POINTS

- Providers caring for intersex patients can ensure *patient centering* when we listen to the goals of care as explained by the patient within the context of what is often a complex and traumatic medical history.
- Crucial for intersex patients is *prevention of further harm*, and providers must understand that many individuals have experienced discrimination and significant harm within healthcare settings; therefore, they have a well-founded mistrust of providers.
- Clinicians must avoid unnecessary questions, unnecessary physical exams, or the urge to ask the patient to teach you about their condition. Understanding the *personal ADLs* of intersex patients means we understand the struggles many intersex patients will face, especially when engaging with healthcare providers. Clinicians must avoid interactions that are invasive or out of our own curiosity, and instead prioritize building trust and providing appropriate care.

CONCLUSION

- Providers lack training and education about the needs of intersex patients.
- Provider biases can alienate intersex patients and their families.
- Providers need to cultivate an understanding of the psychosocial, primary care, and fertility needs of intersex patients.
- Patient-centered care honors patient agency to self-define and mirror patient language.
- The term *intersex* is in current usage and is generally considered favorable to "differences/disorders of sex development."
- The parameters of intersex diagnosis are not medically discreet and patients may use many and varied terms.
- Institutional distrust is common and rooted in the damaging cultural legacy of medical experimentation and nonconsensual medical practices and surgeries.
- Many providers do not recognize, validate, or honor the agency of intersex patients.

Case Study 8.1

Dev is a 14-year-old intersex person coming into the clinic with their parents for gender-affirming care. Dev has been taking estrogen since they were pre-pubertal and were given a genital surgery they were told was necessary for them to have "normal function." Today they come in expressing a lack of understanding about their gender but stating, "I think I'm a man." Dev's parents are expressing support but have a lot of questions.

Considerations: This patient may be accustomed to invasive examinations, while at the same time wary of medical systems. A patient-centered approach involves the clinician listening to the patient's request and validating their experiences, while not asking unnecessary or invasive questions. An invasive physical exam would be unnecessary at the first visit unless requested by the patient; instead, the provider could establish trust with the patient and parents through conversation. The provider could seek to obtain previous medical records to gather more information. If their previous providers were working under the concealment model of care, it is possible the patient and parents may have misunderstanding or lack of information about the physiology or specific intersex states. Since this individual is a minor, and the parents are supportive, coordination of care with the patient, the parents, and an affirming multidisciplinary team will be imperative.

REFERENCES

1. Alpert AB, CichoskiKelly EM, Fox AD. What lesbian, gay, bisexual, transgender, queer, and intersex patients say doctors should know and do: a qualitative study. *J Homosex.* 2017;64(10):1368–1389. doi:10.1080/00918369.2017.1321376

2. Kwok F. The experiences of intersex individuals. The Pitt Pulse. Accessed February 11, 2020. http://www.thepittpulse.org/the-experiences-of-intersex-individuals

3. Frader J, Alderson P, Asch A, et al. Health care professionals and intersex conditions. *Arch Pediatr Adolesc Med.* 2004;158(5):426. doi:10.1001/archpedi.158.5.426

4. Ball J. Cultural safety in practice with children, families and communities. Early Childhood Development Intercultural Partnerships. Accessed November 19, 2019. http://www.ecdip.org/culturalsafety

5. Kellett P, Fitton C. Supporting transvisibility and gender diversity in nursing practice and education: embracing cultural safety. *Nurs Inq.* 2017;24(1):e12146. doi:10.1111/nin.12146

6. Cools M, Robeva R, Hall J, et al. Caring for individuals with a difference of sex development (DSD): a consensus statement. *Nat Rev Endocrinol.* 2018;14(7):415–429. doi:10.1038/s41574-018-0010-8

7. Money J. Imprinting and the establishment of gender role. *Arch Neurol Psychiatr.* 1957;77(3):333. doi:10.1001/archneurpsyc.1957.02330330119019

8. McCann-Crosby B, Mansouri R, Dietrich JE, et al. State of the art review in gonadal dysgenesis: challenges in diagnosis and management. *Int J Pediatr Endocrinol.* 2014;2014(1):4. doi:10.1186/1687-9856-2014-4

9. McCann-Crosby B, Chen M-J, Lyons SK, et al. Nonclassical congenital adrenal hyperplasia: targets of treatment and transition. *Pediatr Endocrinol Rev.* 2014;12(2):224–238. https://pubmed.ncbi.nlm.nih.gov/25581988/

10. Kim KS, Kim J. Disorders of sex development. *Korean J Urol.* 2012;53(1):1. doi:10.4111/kju.2012.53.1.1

11. Kimber CP, Hutson JM. Disorders of sex development (DSD) and laparoscopy. In: Godbole PP, Koyle MA, Wilcox DT, eds. *Pediatric Endourology Techniques.* Springer International Publishing; 2014:183–189. doi:10.1007/978-1-4471-5394-8_20

12. Atta I, Ibrahim M, Parkash A, et al. Etiological diagnosis of undervirilized male/XY disorder of sex development. *J Coll Physicians Surg Pak.* 2014;24:714–718. doi:10.2014/JCPSP.714718

13. MedScape. Androgen excess: practice essentials, pathophysiology, epidemiology. Accessed February 24, 2020. https://emedicine.medscape.com/article/273153-overview#a5

14. Mazza V, Di Monte I, Ceccarelli PL, et al. Prenatal diagnosis of female pseudohermaphroditism associated with bilateral luteoma of pregnancy: case report. *Hum Reprod.* 2002;17(3):821–824. doi:10.1093/humrep/17.3.821

15. Fontana L, Gentilin B, Fedele L, et al. Genetics of Mayer-Rokitansky-Küster-Hauser (MRKH) syndrome: genetics of MRKH syndrome. *Clin Genet.* 2017;91(2):233–246. doi:10.1111/cge.12883

16. Khare J, Deb P, Srivastava P, et al. Swyer syndrome: the gender swayer? *Alex J Med.* 2017;53(2):197–200. doi:10.1016/j.ajme.2016.05.006

17. Mangaraj S, Choudhury A, Mohanty B, et al. Congenital anorchia: a report of two cases and a brief review of the literature. *J Integr Nephro Androl.* 2017;4(4):141. doi:10.4103/jina.jina_4_17

18. Öcal G, Berberoğlu M, Şıklar Z, et al. The clinical and genetic heterogeneity of mixed gonadal dysgenesis: does "disorders of sexual development (DSD)" classification based on new Chicago consensus cover all sex chromosome DSD? *Eur J Pediatr.* 2012;171(10):1497–1502. doi:10.1007/s00431-012-1754-0

19. National Adrenal Diseases Foundation. Congenital adrenal hyperplasia. Accessed February 24, 2020. https://www.nadf.us/congenital-adrenal-hyperplasia-cah.html

20. Genetics Home Reference. Persistent Müllerian duct syndrome. Accessed February 24, 2020. https://ghr.nlm.nih.gov/condition/persistent-mullerian-duct-syndrome
21. American Psychological Association. Answers to your questions about individuals with intersex conditions: (715742007-001). 2006. doi:10.1037/e715742007-001
22. Lee PA, Houk CP, Ahmed SF, et al. Consensus statement on management of intersex disorders. *Pediatrics*. 2006;118(2):e488–e500. doi:10.1542/peds.2006-0738

9

Gender Identity

Dane Menkin, Linda Wesp, Kristin Keglovitz Baker,
Ronica Mukerjee, and Randi Singer

LEARNING OBJECTIVES

By the end of this chapter, the reader will be able to:

- Have a deeper understanding of human gender diversity.
- Conduct a gender affirming intake visit.
- Highlight culturally safe clinical care for transgender, nonbinary, gender nonconforming, and gender expansive patients.
- Utilize evidence-based guidelines for providing gender-affirming hormones and primary care.

INTRODUCTION

Due to the lack of routine data collection of gender identity, demographic information identifying the number of transgender, non-binary, gender non-conforming, and gender expansive* (TGE) people is largely unknown. The Williams Institute estimates 1.4 million or 0.6% of the U.S. population identifies as transgender[1] and all clinicians will care for a person of transgender experience at some point in their career. In order to adequately care for all patients, healthcare providers must be adequately educated to do so. Healthcare providers, however, are largely unprepared for providing care to the transgender population. For example, 80% of gynecologists and 81% of endocrinologists have not received training on the care of transgender patients.[2,3]

---

* The terms *transgender*, *non-binary*, *gender non-conforming*, and *gender expansive* refer to individuals who have a gender identity and/or expression that differ from societal definitions of the gender binary categories that are often assigned at birth based on assigned sex. We will abbreviate using the term "TGE" throughout the chapter to refer to this diverse group of people.

Lack of training around gender-affirming care leads to ambivalence and uncertainty among providers. Research has shown that when providers are uncertain about their ability to provide gender-affirming care, it leads to a fragility of authority and upsets the normal balance of power that we as providers are taught to maintain within the provider-patient relationship.[4] We are learning that when providers are uncertain and ambivalent, we are more likely to act in stigmatizing ways toward transgender patients, perpetuating the cycle of systemic and interpersonal stigma.

Transgender people experience significant barriers to accessing healthcare because of profound levels of explicit and implicit bias and discrimination within healthcare settings.[5–8] The U.S. National Trans Health Survey (USTS) asked respondents about experiences of discrimination healthcare and whether they delayed or avoided seeking care due to fear of discrimination.[5,9] Forty-six percent of respondents reported they experienced discrimination in a previous healthcare encounter.[10] Discrimination in the USTS survey was defined as being denied services, verbally harassed, or physically assaulted. Those who had experienced discrimination were 20 times more likely to report delaying care.[10] A delay of care or avoiding seeking care out of fear of discrimination has been associated with worse health outcomes overall.[11]

Additionally, our transgender patients are facing discrimination and stigma outside of healthcare settings that have lasting implications on health outcomes. For example, 12% of USTS respondents reported being harassed, physically attacked, or sexually assaulted when trying to use a public restroom in the past year.[9] Two-thirds of USTS respondents reported avoiding using the restroom (i.e., "holding it") when they had to urinate, until they could get to a restroom that was private or felt safe. More than 30% of individuals limited the amount they drank to prevent having to use the restroom.

According to a 2018 study that looked at intimate partner violence among young transgender women, self-reports of intimate partner violence were 42% among a cohort of 16- to 24-year-old transgender women in two U.S. cities.[12] The National Coalition of Anti-Violence Programs tracks physical violence, sexual assault, and threats or intimidation across the United States and found that transgender people of color experienced the majority of hate violence incidents out of all reported cases.[12] Additionally, estimates suggest that U.S. Black and Latina transgender women account for nearly 93% of all transgender homicide victims, and that these women are murdered at higher rates than both Black and Latina cisgender women.[13]

Thus, it is imperative that clinicians employ *purposeful self-reflection* and *prevention of harm* in our care for transgender people. Clinicians must regularly assess our level of knowledge and skills as well as any internal biases or discomfort in order to prevent ongoing discrimination and harm in the healthcare setting. We must also understand that transgender people are facing significant victimization throughout their lives.[14] Many resources are available for healthcare providers to increase awareness about the diversity of human gender experiences and expand capacity for providing gender-affirming care. The National LGBT Health Education Center at www.lgbthealtheducation.org has a wide variety of resources including an Implicit Bias Guide for self-assessment and skills building (see Supplemental

Materials available on Springer Connect; visit connect.springerpub.com/content/book/978-0-8261-6921-1 and access the show supplementary dropdown).

OVERVIEW OF GENDER-AFFIRMING CARE

According to the World Professional Association of Transgender Health, gender-affirming medical care can be provided by primary care clinicians, including nurse practitioners, midwives, and physician assistants.[15] Many guidelines exist to offer evidence-based information about doing so (see Table 9.1). Guidelines change regularly, due to an influx in evidence from ongoing research on the long-term effects, dosing, and outcomes of gender-affirming hormone therapy as well as surgeries. We encourage clinicians to incorporate gender-affirming care into their practice by staying updated with evidence-based guidelines and by engaging in regular, purposeful self-reflection to ensure high-quality and gender-affirming care. In general, primary care for transgender people is not different from routine primary care. Individuals on hormone therapy should receive the same routine prevention and screening, with several minor exceptions discussed in the text that follows under Cancer Screening Considerations.

The guidelines in Table 9.1 are recommended references for the most up-to-date practices including primary care, hormone dosing, laboratory monitoring, and surgery guidelines.

TABLE 9.1 Evidence-Based Guidelines for Gender Affirming Care

Lyon Martin Health Services: Project Health TransLine	project-health.org/transline
University of California San Francisco Center of Excellence for Transgender Health: Guidelines for the primary and gender-affirming care of transgender and gender nonbinary people	transcare.ucsf.edu/guidelines
Endocrine Society: Endocrine treatment of gender-dysphoric/gender-incongruent persons: an Endocrine Society Clinical Practice Guideline	academic.oup.com/jcem/article/102/11/3869/4157558#99603237
Sherbourne Health: Guidelines and Protocols for Hormone Therapy and Primary Health Care for Trans Clients	www.rainbowhealthontario.ca/TransHealthGuide
National Organization of Nurse Practitioner Faculties: Patient-Centered Transgender Health	cdn.ymaws.com/www.nonpf.org/resource/resmgr/files/transgender_toolkit_final.pdf
World Professional Association for Transgender Health standards of care (Version 8 due out in 2020, which will include expanded primary care recommendations)	www.wpath.org

GENDER-AFFIRMING INTAKE AND REVIEW OF SYSTEMS

We encourage a review of Chapter 2 on Language and Communication to ensure gender-affirming approaches throughout the patient visit. A gender-affirming patient intake will include sensitivity to the *personal activities of daily living (ADLs)* that individuals engage in to ensure safety and affirmation throughout their daily lives. When meeting someone for the first time, clinicians should also be mindful to remain *patient centered* and *prevent harm*. Given the likelihood that transgender patients have previously experienced discrimination in the healthcare setting, establishing trust may take time. The following points should be considered as components of a comprehensive intake for transgender/gender expansive (TGE) people in the general primary care setting. The first step of an intake visit is to understand the patient's goals. Additional detailed information can be gathered over multiple visits. Here are some topics that may be covered with some suggestions for language you may want to adopt for your practice:

1.   If the patient is coming to establish care for gender-affirming interventions, such as hormones or referrals for surgery, the first and most important topic of discussion should be a thorough discussion about the patient's goals. Open-ended questions can begin the conversation, and evidence-based information can also be provided if the provider is looking to obtain more information. *Partnerships* between provider and patient can be established during this first visit as patient goals are explored. *"What are your goals for today's visit?"* If coming to establish care for hormones: *"What are your goals and desires for hormone therapy? What questions do you have?"*

2.   Current and past hormone use (names/doses of medications, administration method, history of time on or off hormone therapy, and if prescribed by a licensed physician or through their own means). *"Do you currently take any medication, vitamins, or use over-the-counter or non-prescribed medications regularly?"*

3.   Surgical history and an accurate documentation of organs present to guide primary care screenings and acute care evaluation. Using patient's preferred terminology for body parts or general terms is recommended. *"I have some questions about your body and any history of surgeries." "How do you prefer to refer to your body parts?" "Have you had any gender-affirming surgeries?"*

4.   The practice of other gender-affirming interventions such as binding of breasts, tucking of genitals, use of injectable silicone or other filler substances, hair removal procedures such as laser or electrolysis, or hair loss prevention interventions. *For trans masculine patients: "Do you use a binder? If so, do you have any issues or concerns about binding?" For trans feminine patients: "Do you tuck or use a gaff? Do you do any laser or electrolysis for hair removal?" "Have you ever used silicone or other fillers?"*

5.   Sexual history to assess and discuss desires around planning/prevention of pregnancy, HIV/STI testing/proactive prevention (see Chapter 10 for detailed information). *"Are you sexually active?" "What are your sexual practices?"* or *"What body parts come in contact with partners when you have sex? Do you use your front or back for sex? Both?" "When were you last screened for HIV and other STDs?"*

6. Social history including trauma-informed assessment of previous experiences of rejection, victimization, abuse among family, intimate partners, school, employment, or housing. *"Does anyone put their hands on you in a way which scares or hurts you or is unwanted?" "Does anyone in your house yell, scream or scare you or anyone else in the house?" "Have you been in a situation where a person has told you they love you but they also hit you or make you ashamed?"*

Clearly, we all develop our own style when it comes to talking with patients. Dialogue that affirms gender identity while obtaining essential information is crucial for providing patient-specific care. The examples of language have been provided for consideration, and we encourage clinicians to practice and develop their own gender-affirming approach so they are comfortable in their conversation with people, as this is also crucial for developing trust.

LANGUAGE TIPS FOR INTAKE INTERVIEW WITH TRANSGENDER PATIENTS

The following are some tips by the authors of this chapter, all practicing clinicians and gender-affirming hormone prescribers.

"So ... about the people you connect with for sex or play. ... Are they people with penises/without penises? Do you use their parts down below for sex/play? And, do you use condoms for oral, front hole, and/or back hole?" [Dane Menkin, FNP]

"Many people have already done a lot of research about changes from gender-affirming hormones before they come in to see me for the first time. What are some changes you are desiring? Are there any questions you have about hormones that we could address right away? Would you be comfortable sharing if you have any specific goals for hormone therapy?" [Linda Wesp, FNP]

PHYSICAL EXAM

Gender-Affirming Physical Exam

Physical examination should be relevant to the present anatomy, regardless of gender presentation, and without assumptions as to anatomy or identity. Providers should use a gender-affirming approach when conducting a physical exam. This includes referring to the patient by their correct name and pronouns during the entire visit. When explaining the physical exam either prior to or during examination, clinicians should again use the patient's preferred terminology for specific body parts rather than traditional medical terminology like "penis" or "breasts." A transmasculine individual, for example, may be uncomfortable with terms such as *vulva*, *vagina*, or *clitoris*. In this case, we must be confident asking patients what terms they use when referring to various parts of their body).[16] Oftentimes, people use front hole or back hole. Additionally, as with all patients, examinations should only be performed on the body parts that pertain to the reason for the visit. For example, there is no reason to assess the genitals of someone being seen for otitis media.

Binding of the chest to create a masculine appearance may lead to skin breakdown or other complications of the skin, as well as musculoskeletal pain or changes in posture.[17] Similarly, tucking penis and testicles to create a more feminine appearance may cause irritation to the meatus, discomfort in the scrotal area, or skin conditions such as tinea cruris. Patients may be hesitant to remove the binder or gaff for a physical exam, and *patient-centered* care can be provided by discussing the concerning symptom. Obtaining a history alone may be what is needed for a patient to try a treatment measure. Some patients may wish to come back at a different time for a physical exam or wait to see if the symptoms improve.

Secondary sex characteristics may be noticeable on physical exam in patients undergoing hormone therapy, depending on duration of hormone use and age of initiation (see Tables 9.2 and 9.3). Transmasculine people may have facial and body hair growth, clitoromegaly, increased muscle mass, masculine fat redistribution, androgenic alopecia, and acne.[18] Transfeminine people will experience gradual feminine fat redistribution and breast development. The development of breast tissue often occurs with an increase in nipple sensitivity and a palpable lump or "breast bud." This

TABLE 9.2 Effects of Testosterone

EFFECT OF TESTOSTERONE	EXPECTED ONSET	EXPECTED MAXIMUM EFFECT	REVERSIBILITY IF TESTOSTERONE STOPPED
Facial/body hair growth	3–6 months	1–5 years	Irreversible
Increased muscle mass/strength (significantly dependent on amount of exercise)	6–12 months	1–5 years	Reversible
Deepened voice	3–12 months	1–2 years	Irreversible
Cessation of menstrual periods	2–6 months	n/a	Reversible
Clitoral enlargement (by 1–3 cm)	3–6 months	1–2 years	Irreversible
Body fat redistribution to a more masculine pattern (decreased on buttocks/hips/thighs, increased in abdomen)	3–6 months	2–5 years	Reversible
Skin oiliness/acne (may be severe)	1–6 months	1–2 years	Reversible
Scalp hair loss (temples and crown of head, highly dependent on age and inheritance)	Variable	Variable	Irreversible
Increased libido	Variable	Variable	Reversible

Source: Data from Endocrine Society. Hembree WC, Cohen-Kettenis PT, Gooren L, et al. Endocrine treatment of gender-dysphoric/gender-incongruent persons: an Endocrine Society Clinical Practice Guideline. *J Clin Endocrinol Metabol.* 2017;102(11):3869–3903. doi:10.1210/jc.2017-01658.

TABLE 9.3 Effects of Estrogen/Anti-androgens

EFFECT OF ESTROGEN/ ANTI-ANDROGEN	EXPECTED ONSET OF EFFECT	EXPECTED MAXIMUM EFFECT	REVERSIBILITY IF ESTROGEN/ANTI- ANDROGEN IS STOPPED
Breast growth	3–6 months	2–3 years	Irreversible
Thinning/slowed growth of body and facial hair	6–12 months	3–5 years	Reversible
Softening of skin/decreased oiliness	3–6 months	Variable	Reversible
Body fat redistribution (increased on buttocks/hips/ thighs/chest, decreased in abdomen)	3–6 months	2–5 years	Reversible
Decreased muscle mass/ strength	3–6 months	1–2 years	Reversible
Decreased libido	1–3 months	1–2 years	Reversible
Decreased spontaneous erections	1–3 months	3–6 months	Reversible
Male sexual dysfunction (e.g., erections not as firm)	Variable	Variable	Reversible
Decreased sperm production/maturation, reduced fertility	variable	variable	Possibly Irreversible
Decreased testicular volume	3–6 months	2–3 years	Likely irreversible
Cessation of male pattern balding	No regrowth, loss stops 1–3 months	1–2 years	Reversible

Source: Data from Endocrine Society. Hembree WC, Cohen-Kettenis PT, Gooren L, et al. Endocrine treatment of gender-dysphoric/gender-incongruent persons: an Endocrine Society Clinical Practice Guideline. *J Clin Endocrinol Metabol.* 2017;102(11):3869–3903. doi:10.1210/jc.2017-01658.

breast development mirrors that of cisgender female puberty including the need for supportive undergarments.

Patients who have undergone gender-affirming surgeries may have varying physical exam findings depending on the procedures performed, approaches used, and occurrence of complications.

Special Considerations for Pelvic Exam in Transgender Women

Transgender women who have had vaginoplasty will have specific anatomy that is important to be aware of. The neovagina created through the most commonly performed penile-inversion technique is not a mucosal membrane, but rather squamous cell tissue. Patients will be instructed to dilate daily to maintain the vaginal girth and depth. The vaginal canal ends in a blind cuff that lacks a cervix or surrounding fornices. The vaginal opening may be more posterior and the prostate is not removed during surgery, and the prostate can be found at the anterior vaginal wall. If visualization of the neovagina is required, use of an anoscope may provide better visualization.[15,19]

The anatomy of a neovagina created in a transgender woman differs from a natal vagina in that it is a blind cuff, lacks a cervix or surrounding fornices, and may have a more posterior orientation. As such, using an anoscope may be a more anatomically appropriate approach for a visual examination. The anoscope can be inserted, the trocar removed, and the vaginal walls visualized collapsing around the end of the anoscope as it is withdrawn.

Special Considerations for Pelvic Exam in Transgender Men

Special considerations for the pelvic exam are important for transmasculine clients. A pelvic or genital exam may be a traumatic and anxiety-inducing procedure for transgender men and other transmasculine persons due to gender dysphoria or previous negative experiences with providers. A bimanual exam or speculum exam can be made less uncomfortable when the provider is thoughtful in the approach, and uses patient-centered decision-making. Discussing procedures beforehand, including what will be needed and why, is an essential component of culturally safe care. Discussion beforehand allows the patient to express any concerns, and offers care providers the opportunity to address these concerns. Creating a safe space for patients who do choose to proceed with an exam can include inviting the patient to have a support person in the room or listen to music on headphones. For those with severe anxiety, an oral benzodiazepine 20 to 60 minutes prior to the exam has been successful.[20]

Communication techniques during the procedure are essential.[21,22] Some patients may want to know exactly what is happening (when they will feel a touch, when the clicking of the speculum will occur, and so on) while others may want to talk about something entirely unrelated or have silence. Inquiring what is best for each individual is essential. Additionally, assure the patient that the exam can be stopped at any time at their request and then stop immediately if the patient asks. Some providers offer a mirror so the patient can directly observe what is happening; however, some patients may find this offensive and it may contribute to dysphoria.

If vaginal atrophy is significant, due to continuous testosterone use, vaginal estrogens can be used for several weeks prior to attempting to repeat the exam.[23] Self-collection of vaginal swabs for HPV or vaginitis evaluation are also appropriate, and may prevent the need for a speculum exam.[7]

CANCER SCREENING CONSIDERATIONS

In general, data about long-term effects of hormone therapy are lacking. Current best practices are based on expert opinion and available research. The general rule for cancer screening is to remain aware of what organs are present in your patient and conduct education and screening as appropriate according to national guidelines for the general population. Clinicians should keep in mind that patient education materials and provider language about "self-breast exams" or "self-testicular exams" may require updating so they maintain a culturally safe *partnership* and *patient-centered* approach. Obtaining history as it pertains to genetic cancer risk is important in the areas of reproductive organs such as breast or ovarian cancer. Referral for genetic screening should follow evidence-based guidelines for individuals with ovaries and breasts. Several other specific considerations are outlined in the text that follows for transmasculine and transfeminine patients.

Transmasculine People

Primary care considerations for transmasculine people should include an awareness about the history of hormone use, and then proceed with routine screening as per current national guidelines depending on the body parts present. In a 2015 study conducted by the National Center for Transgender Equality, 22% of transgender people did not wish to seek gender-affirming hormones and 27% of trans men didn't want chest reduction, often referred to as "top" surgery.[9]

While the majority of the healthcare needs for the transmasculine patient are similar to any patient, a few things stand out as specific needs. If the patient still has organs that could develop reproductive cancers (i.e., uterus, ovaries, cervix, breasts), screening at intervals should take place as they regularly would per the age-based preventative care guidelines. Routine ovarian and endometrial cancer screening is not conducted for the general population, and evidence is lacking to indicate that testosterone therapy has any differential impact on risk. Breast cancer screening should follow national guidelines if the patient has not had chest masculinization surgery.[24] Note that chest masculinization surgery does not remove all breast tissue, but does reduce the chest to a masculine appearance whereby mammography would not be an option for screening purposes. Self-chest exams or clinical exams can ascertain and evaluate abnormalities, and ultrasound can be conducted to evaluated abnormal masses.[25]

Cervical cancer screening is recommended for all people with a cervix according to national guidelines. However, individuals with a cervix on testosterone therapy have atrophic changes to the cervix and vagina, which can result in high numbers of "inadequate cells" for cytology results.[14] Research is underway to examine the option of self-collected HPV-only screening (i.e., no pathology sample collected using a speculum). When cytology is collected, it is essential to make clear to the laboratory that the sample being provided is indeed a cervical Pap smear (especially if the listed gender marker is "male") to avoid the sample being run incorrectly as an anal pap or discarded. The use of testosterone or presence of amenorrhea should also be indicated on the requisition. Should the individual express distress or concern about the examination, it may be deferred until a later date once a trusting relationship has been developed.

Transfeminine People

Transgender women on estrogen therapy will develop breast tissue that reaches maximum growth at about 3 to 5 years. Breast cancer is very likely less prevalent among transgender women compared to cisgender women, especially if hormone therapy was started after puberty, due to less overall lifetime exposure to estrogen. Several retrospective studies suggest lower risk of breast cancer among transgender women compared to cisgender women.[26,27] Transgender women do have more dense breasts and some individuals may have breast implants, which is important to take into consideration because both can lower the accuracy of mammography.[28,29]

Because of the dearth of research-based evidence, current best practices about when to start conducting mammograms for transgender women is based on expert opinion. It is recommended to defer screening mammogram for individuals who otherwise meet age requirements until the individual has been on estrogen therapy for at least 5 years because of the length of time it takes for breast tissue to develop. Providers should refer to currently published guidelines for any changes to this practice, based on new evidence.

Clinicians should also keep in mind that transgender women who have had vaginoplasty will retain their prostate. As previously mentioned, it will be located anteriorly to the neovagina. Prostate exam would then be most accurately performed with a digital vaginal exam focused on the anterior aspect of the vaginal canal.[30] Prostate cancer screening guidelines for the general population should be followed; however, it is important to note that transgender women will likely be of much lower risk due to lower overall lifetime exposure to testosterone. Several cases of prostate cancer have been documented in the literature, and may present with otherwise asymptomatic hematuria.[31-33]

Transfeminine people on estrogen therapy will experience a decrease in testicular volume, and overall lower lifetime exposure to testosterone theoretically reduces the risk for testicular cancer. Long-term evidence about risk is lacking. Routine testicular cancer screening does not exist for the general population outside of testicular self-exams, which may be uncomfortable or cause dysphoria among transfeminine people. One case report of testicular cancer has been reported in the literature, suggesting that clinicians should be aware of abnormal findings and evaluate accordingly.[34]

Case Studies 9.1 and 9.2 will provide the reader the opportunity to apply skills learned in this chapter.

Case Study 9.1: Dale

Dale, a 24-year-old trans guy on masculinizing hormones for over 10 years, calls your office Monday morning after presenting to urgent care on Saturday with dysuria and urinary frequency. He reports having tried to "drink a lot of water to see if it would help" but his symptoms continue to worsen so he went to urgent care. Dale's medical history includes the diagnosis of gender dysphoria and anxiety. His only medication is testosterone. He reports this "happened to me a long time ago and it turned out to be a bladder infection." Dale identified himself as a transgender male to the urgent care provider and his wife was with him.

(continued)

Dale reports he provided a urine sample and was told that most urinary tract infections in men are a result of sexually transmitted infections; therefore, it was suggested that he be tested for HIV and syphilis. Dale offered that he and his wife are monogamous partners of over 5 years and that an STD was quite unlikely, and he declined the further STD testing. The clinician then asked why such a young man was taking testosterone; again, Dale explained he is a transgender male and needs hormones to sustain his transition.

Dale declined the STI testing and was informed by the clinician that it is suspected that he either has an STI or that the testosterone is causing his symptoms and they advised he stop taking them. Dale was provided with a referral to a urologist. Dale didn't feel this was correct so he left and called your office first thing Monday morning. He woke up feeling nauseated with fever and chills today, with continued dysuria and frequency. He noticed blood in his urine as well this morning.

CASE DISCUSSION

Dale has experienced inappropriate care by another healthcare provider, and has symptoms that have worsened because he received inadequate evaluation and treatment for urinary symptoms that were consistent with a UTI or bladder infection. The urgent care provider was distracted and uninformed about Dale's hormone therapy and did not listen to his personal sexual history—and inappropriately assumed the symptoms were a sexually transmitted infection and something related to the testosterone. (*Note:* Testosterone therapy does not have any known adverse effects related to dysuria or UTIs.) Dale is now having worsening symptoms that indicate possible pyelonephritis due to poor clinical judgment. Furthermore, the visit in urgent care was not patient centered, culturally safe, or gender affirming. Instead of preventing harm, the clinician's ineptitude contributed to the patient's worsening physical symptoms and psychological distress.

As Dale's primary care provider, you are aware that testosterone does not cause UTIs. You listen to Dale's report of his sexual history, and agree it is unlikely his symptoms are an STI. You are aware of the possibility that transmasculine people may experience discrimination when using public restrooms, and often have had experiences of having to hold it or restrict fluids because it is unsafe to go to the bathroom when in public spaces.

Dale is added into your schedule for Monday and upon arrival you check a urine dipstick which indicates a urinary tract or bladder infection. Dale is afebrile and no longer nauseous, but continues to notice blood in his urine and has dysuria and frequency. You proceed accordingly for testing and treatment of a bladder infection. As you talk further with Dale about the history, you learn that he was at a music festival for an entire day and because he was uncomfortable using the festival restroom, he restricted his fluids and didn't void for 10 hours.

Case Study 9.2: Kay

Kay is a 22-year-old African American transgender woman. She has been taking hormones and anti-androgens for medical transition for over 10 years and had a vaginoplasty 4 years ago. Kay's driver's license states her first name is Christopher with a gender marker of "male" but her insurance card has Kay as her legal first name and her gender as female. Her last name and date of birth are the same on both forms of ID.

Kay presents to the ED with a 3-inch long laceration above her left eyebrow and noted bruising around her left eye as well as a swollen lip. Her pants have a tear in them and her belt is broken. She is accompanied by a person she identifies as her sister but the relationship is questioned by the registrar.

Kay tells the triage nurse in the ED that she is taking estrogen 2 mg tablets twice daily and Truvada. She reports she fell off the curb a few hours ago while trying to cross the street. She says she hit her head on the curb when she fell and "thinks she needs stitches."

Upon admission to the ED, Kay's friend is asked to wait in the ED waiting room, and someone will come get her shortly. Kay asks to have her stay with her but is advised that it is policy to not have visitors in the ED. Kay is seen by the resident and tells her the same story of the injury that she had told the triage nurse. The resident asks why a woman her age would take estrogen and asks "Is that birth control?" Kay tells the resident she is a transgender woman and explains that the estrogen is what she takes for her transition. She explains that she takes the Truvada to protect herself from getting HIV if she is exposed to it through a partner.

The resident asks for a urine sample and explains that it is needed to look for "substances which could have contributed to her fall." Kay explains she had not been drinking or using any drugs and declines to leave the urine sample. Kay's sister is allowed back after about an hour and sits with her in the room. The sister discloses to the nurse privately that she is worried Kay was assaulted and in fact did not fall. She asks if there was maybe a social worker or special nurse who could come talk to her. She is worried she might have also been sexually assaulted and should be offered testing. The nurse tells her Kay had refused the urine sample so they can't do anything else except suture her laceration. The head laceration is sutured by the resident, and her facial wounds are treated. Kay is discharged from the ED with Ibuprofen for her headache and instructions to return if her headache worsens.

CASE DISCUSSION

This case is an example of why patients hesitate to disclose a transgender identity or use of gender-affirming hormones. The clinician's lack of knowledge about transgender care led to his assumption about estradiol being used for birth control. Clinician discomfort may have led to stigmatizing interactions throughout the visit. Too often, a transgender person who presents for care of an illness or

(continued)

injury is treated as if their trans identity is relevant to the presenting concern. Otherwise, their disclosure of trans status can distract from the true issue at hand and create unnecessary scrutiny. It seems quite obvious to any clinician reading this case that the injuries sustained by Kay are inconsistent with the described mechanism of injury. In this case, the initiation of testing for substances relays the message of distrust and disbelief, automatically leaving Kay further isolated when she may need further resources for safety. Despite the efforts of the sister, the clinicians missed opportunities for building trust and providing more complete and thorough care that addressed glaring safety needs.

CULTURAL SAFETY SUMMARY POINTS

- We can employ *purposeful self-reflection* in our care of transgender and gender expansive patients to create a safe experience during healthcare encounters: start with assessing your level of knowledge and skills, as well as any discomfort you notice when caring for TGE people.
- *Prevention of harm* can include ongoing education about language, communication, and best practices for providing evidence-based care to TGE populations. Many resources exist but you can start with bookmarking the list of sources in Table 9.1 for regular referencing.
- Set aside time to work through the National LGBT Health Education Center's Implicit Bias Guide (see Supplemental Materials available on Springer Connect; visit connect.springerpub.com/content/book/978-0-8261-6921-1 and access the show supplementary dropdown) and other trainings. Encourage all colleagues in your practice to complete these as well. Ongoing education will expand your understanding of the harmful experiences your patient may have had in healthcare settings. Collaboration with others will create systems allowing for *patient centering* and clinician knowledge about the *personal ADLs* your patients may be experiencing.
- A gender-affirming patient intake will include sensitivity to the *personal activities of daily living (ADLs)* that individuals engage in to ensure safety and affirmation throughout their daily lives. A first step is to understand patient goals for seeking care, using open-ended questions and building trust by approaching care through the framework of *patient partnerships*.

CONCLUSION

In order to provide culturally safe care for all of our patients, we must meet them where they are. We must look past the name on the insurance card and ask open-ended questions without assuming what answers may follow. By mirroring a patients' preferred language in relation to body parts or pronouns, we are honoring their human dignity. When we treat our patients respectfully and provide gender-affirming care, we begin to earn our patient's trust. This foundation of trust and mutual respect paves the way for holistic, evidence-based, and patient-centered care.

REFERENCES

1. Flores AR, Herman JL, Gates GJ, et al. *How Many Adults Identify as Transgender in the United States?* Williams Institute; 2016.
2. Davidge-Pitts C, Nippoldt TB, Danoff A, et al. Transgender health in endocrinology: current status of endocrinology fellowship programs and practicing clinicians. *J Clin Endocrinol Metab.* 2017;102(4):1286–1290. doi:10.1210/jc.2016-3007
3. Unger CA. Care of the transgender patient: a survey of gynecologists' current knowledge and practice. *J Womens Health.* 2015;24(2):114–118. doi:10.1089/jwh.2014.4918
4. Poteat T, German D, Kerrigan D. Managing uncertainty: a grounded theory of stigma in transgender health care encounters. *Soc Sci Med.* 2013;84:22–29. doi:10.1016/j.socscimed.2013.02.019
5. Grant JM, Mottet L, Tanis J, et al. *Injustice at Every Turn: A Report of the National Transgender Discrimination Survey.* National Center for Transgender Equality; 2011.
6. Cruz TM. Assessing access to care for transgender and gender nonconforming people: a consideration of diversity in combating discrimination. *Soc Sci Med.* 2014;110:65–73. doi:10.1016/j.socscimed.2014.03.032
7. Rodriguez A, Agardh A, Asamoah BO. Self-reported discrimination in health-care settings based on recognizability as transgender: a cross-sectional study among transgender U.S. citizens. *Arch Sex Behav.* 2018;47(4):973–985. doi:10.1007/s10508-017-1028-z
8. Kcomt L. Profound health-care discrimination experienced by transgender people: rapid systematic review. *Soc Work Health Care.* 2019;58(2):201–219. doi:10.1080/00981389.2018.1532941
9. James S, Herman JL, Rankin S, et al. *The Report of the 2015 U.S. Transgender Survey.* National Center for Transgender Equality; 2016.
10. Glick JL, Theall KP, Andrinopoulos KM, et al. The role of discrimination in care postponement among trans-feminine individuals in the U.S. National Transgender Discrimination Survey. *LGBT Health.* 2018;5(3):171–179. doi:10.1089/lgbt.2017.0093
11. Seelman KL, Colón-Diaz MJP, LeCroix RH, et al. Transgender noninclusive healthcare and delaying care because of fear: connections to general health and mental health among transgender adults. *Transgender Health.* 2017;2(1):17–28. doi:10.1089/trgh.2016.0024
12. Garthe RC, Hidalgo MA, Hereth J, et al. Prevalence and risk correlates of intimate partner violence among a multisite cohort of young transgender women. *LGBT Health.* 2018;5(6):333–340. doi:10.1089/lgbt.2018.0034
13. Dinno A. Homicide rates of transgender individuals in the United States: 2010–2014. *Am J Public Health.* 2017;107(9):1441–1447. doi:10.2105/AJPH.2017.303878
14. Reisner SL, Hughto JMW, Dunham EE, et al. Legal protections in public accommodations settings: a critical public health issue for transgender and gender-nonconforming people: protecting transgender people in public accommodations. *Milbank Q.* 2015;93(3):484–515. doi:10.1111/1468-0009.12127
15. Coleman E, Bockting W, Botzer M, et al. Standards of care for the health of transsexual, transgender, and gender-nonconforming people, version 7. *Int J Transgenderism.* 2012;13(4):165–232. doi:10.1080/15532739.2011.700873
16. Dutton L, Koenig K, Fennie K. Gynecologic care of the female-to-male transgender man. *J Midwifery Womens Health.* 2008;53:331–337. doi:10.1016/j.jmwh.2008.02.003
17. Peitzmeier S, Gardner I, Weinand J, et al. Health impact of chest binding among transgender adults: a community-engaged, cross-sectional study. *Cult Health Sex.* 2017;19(1):64–75. doi:10.1080/13691058.2016.1191675

18. Feldman J, Goldberg J. Transgender primary medical care. *Int J Transgend*. 2006;9:3–34. doi:10.1300/J485v09n03_02

19. Transgender Care. Transgender people and sexually transmitted infections (STIs). Accessed February 4, 2020. https://transcare.ucsf.edu/guidelines/stis

20. Eckstrand KL, Potter J, Edmiston EK. Obstetric and gynecologic care for individuals who are LGBT. In: Eckstrand K, Ehrenfeld JM, eds. *Lesbian, Gay, Bisexual, and Transgender Healthcare: A Clinical Guide to Preventive, Primary, and Specialist Care*. Springer International Publishing; 2016:309–336. doi:10.1007/978-3-319-19752-4_17

21. Bonvicini KA, Perlin MJ. The same but different: clinician–patient communication with gay and lesbian patients. *Patient Educ Couns*. 2003;51(2):115–122. doi:10.1016/S0738-3991(02)00189-1

22. Goins ES, Pye D. Check the box that best describes you: reflexively managing theory and praxis in LGBTQ health communication research. *Health Commun*. 2013;28(4):397–407. doi:10.1080/10410236.2012.690505

23. Peitzmeier SM, Reisner SL, Harigopal P, et al. Female-to-male patients have high prevalence of unsatisfactory Paps compared to non-transgender females: implications for cervical cancer screening. *J Gen Intern Med*. 2014;29(5):778–784. doi:10.1007/s11606-013-2753-1

24. US Preventive Services Task Force. Breast Cancer Screening Guidelines. Accessed February 4, 2020. https://www.uspreventiveservicestaskforce.org/uspstf/recommendation/breast-cancer-screening

25. Siu AL, on behalf of the U.S. Preventive Services Task Force. Screening for breast cancer: U.S. Preventive Services Task Force recommendation statement. *Ann Intern Med*. 2016;164(4):279. doi:10.7326/M15-2886

26. Brown GR, Jones KT. Incidence of breast cancer in a cohort of 5,135 transgender veterans. *Breast Cancer Res Treat*. 2015;149(1):191–198. doi:10.1007/s10549-014-3213-2

27. Asscheman H, Giltay EJ, Megens JAJ, et al. A long-term follow-up study of mortality in transsexuals receiving treatment with cross-sex hormones. *Eur J Endocrinol*. 2011;164(4):635–642. doi:10.1530/EJE-10-1038

28. Weyers S, Villeirs G, Vanherreweghe E, et al. Mammography and breast sonography in transsexual women. *Eur J Radiol*. 2010;74(3):508–513. doi:10.1016/j.ejrad.2009.03.018

29. Gooren LJ, van Trotsenburg MAA, Giltay EJ, et al. Breast cancer development in transsexual subjects receiving cross-sex hormone treatment. *J Sex Med*. 2013;10(12):3129–3134. doi:10.1111/jsm.12319

30. Transgender Care. Prostate and testicular cancer considerations in transgender women. Accessed February 6, 2020. https://transcare.ucsf.edu/guidelines/prostate-testicular-cancer

31. Miksad RA, Bubley G, Church P, et al. Prostate cancer in a transgender woman 41 years after initiation of feminization. *JAMA*. 2006;296(19):2316–2317. doi:10.1001/jama.296.19.2316

32. Turo R, Jallad S, Prescott S, et al. Metastatic prostate cancer in transsexual diagnosed after three decades of estrogen therapy. *Can Urol Assoc J*. 2013;7(7–8):E544–546. doi:10.5489/cuaj.175

33. Dorff TB, Shazer RL, Nepomuceno EM, et al. Successful treatment of metastatic androgen-independent prostate carcinoma in a transsexual patient. *Clin Genitourin Cancer*. 2007;5(5):344–346. doi:10.3816/CGC.2007.n.016

34. Wolf-Gould CS, Wolf-Gould CH. A transgender woman with testicular cancer: a new twist on an old problem. *LGBT Health*. 2016;3(1):90–95. doi:10.1089/lgbt.2015.0057

Specific Approaches to Care

Sexual Healthcare for LGBTQIA+ Individuals

Linda Wesp, Danielle Boudreau, Ronica Mukerjee, and Lazarus Nance Letcher

LEARNING OBJECTIVES

By the end of this chapter, the reader will be able to:

- Discuss three ways to take a culturally safe sexual health history.
- Identify options for providing a trauma-informed pelvic exam.
- Discuss three ways to support sexual function and pleasure for all patients.
- Describe screening recommendations for sexually transmitted infections.

INTRODUCTION

Sexual health is a fluctuating state of well-being that encompasses the physical, emotional, psychological, and possibly spiritual aspects of one's sexual experience. Sexual health is fluid, individual, and evolving based on a person's experience in any given moment in time.[1] Sexuality includes a constellation of experiences, which can be expressed in a variety of ways with shifts and evolution over time.[2] The clinician's role in supporting a person's sexual health is to individualize the counseling and care provided based on the patient's communicated experiences and preferences. There are no prescriptive or "cookie-cutter" approaches based on an individual's sexuality, gender identity, or sexual expression and behavior. This chapter is intended to provide clinicians with some fundamental knowledge and tools to begin customizing their communication skills and approach to care in order to meet each patient's unique needs.

Sexuality is heavily stigmatized in American society (for more detailed discussion see Chapter 3).[3] Stigma multiplies for individuals who have what are perceived to be "deviant" bodies by the dominant cisgender-heteronormative-ableist narratives.[4,5] Individuals with fat bodies, black and brown bodies, queer and trans bodies, and differently abled bodies are all confronted with varying levels of stigma and ignorance.[4,6,7] Deep cultural narratives exist which assert that an individual's worth is tied up in their sexual choices, potency, and/or level of sexual appeal.[3,8,9] There is a concerted effort to mediate and commodify sexuality through the dieting industry, hair dyes and relaxants, clothing made to hide fat composition, and teeth whiteners. The commodification of the idealized sexual form serves to propagate vast disparities which benefit white, thin, able-bodied, cisgender, heteronormative people and further marginalize those who are black/brown, fat, queer, trans, and differently abled. The impacts that these narratives can have on the physical and mental health of those who own a "deviant" body can be profound.[10]

Sexual health and desire can manifest as healthy self-expression, connection with others, stress reduction, and pleasure.[1,2] Separating sexual expression from reproduction or family planning is essential. In this chapter we will explore concepts of stigma, shame, and bodily autonomy grounded in frameworks of cultural safety, trauma-informed care, and social justice. At its heart, this chapter is about listening. We trust that our patients have the answers and know what is best for themselves. At our best, clinicians can be instrumental in removing the burden the patient may feel in educating their clinician about their sexual health, while providing the clinician with tools to support the goals patients identify for themselves.

TAKING A SEXUAL HEALTH HISTORY

Individual sexuality manifests in many ways. Sexual expression, sexual behavior, and pleasure are all components of sexual intimacy and impact sexual health.[1,2] Although not the focus of this chapter, asexuality is also a normal variant and healthy relationship to sexuality, and is discussed in greater detail in Chapter 7.[11-13] Cultural norms assume that "having sex" means insertive penile-vaginal intercourse. First, clinicians must recognize that this culturally assumed definition of "having sex" is far from true. Next, clinicians must be knowledgeable about the complex nature of sexuality and use this to inform communication with patients, especially LGBTQIA+ populations who have experienced marginalization due to these cultural norms and inaccurate assumptions.[14]

A tailored approach to sexual health screening, advice, and care requires that care providers understand an individual's sexual behavior.[15] Sharing details about sexual practices may feel uncomfortable or unsafe for individuals who have been previously shamed by society at large. Why would someone choose to disclose details about their sexuality when they have been previously discriminated against, or judged about their sexual behavior by a healthcare provider?[16] Therefore, the authors of this text recommend beginning an intake about sexual history with a statement such as "As a component of your overall holistic healthcare, I have a few questions for you about your sexual health that I ask all of my patients." To create an environment of trust and understanding, follow-up statements should acknowledge that the discussion is not mandatory and may be discussed at a future time if the patient does not want to address these issues today.

Clinicians must be aware that sexual behavior may exist within myriad of relationship structures, including monogamy, consensual non-monogamy or polyamory, sex in exchange for money or goods, or BDSM/kink play (see Chapter 6 for more information).[17] A nonjudgmental approach to sexual healthcare is crucial to ascertain pertinent information. Clinicians can remember the 5 Ps for a comprehensive sexual history: Past STIs, Pregnancy plans and history, sexual Practices, sexual Partners, and Prevention of STIs/HIV.[18]

At the crux of understanding sexual practices is gathering information from the patient about the use of sex toys and which body parts go where with another person. Oftentimes, questions about sexual practices can be connected to conversations about available screenings and associated risks. Offering information without eliciting immediate response allows the individual to decide what they may be at risk for based on their previous experiences.

For example, when offering HIV, gonorrhea/chlamydia, and syphilis testing, the clinician can discuss the ways these infections are spread. Since HIV is spread through four main bodily fluids (semen/ejaculate, vaginal secretions, blood, and breastmilk), it would be important to understand whether and how often the patient has experienced direct contact (minus a barrier such as a condom) of another's bodily fluids to their susceptible body parts. This might include having a penis inside their vagina/genital canal or anus, or inserting their penis inside a vagina/genital canal or anus. For gonorrhea and chlamydia, if an individual only ever receives a penis into their mouth but never has any other contact with other parts of their body, their throat may be the only potential site of infection with either of these bacteria. A urine test will not accurately detect gonorrhea and chlamydia if the only potential site of infection is the throat.

Intake questions may also involve asking about signs or symptoms, which may be disclosed only after enough trust is established in the provider-patient relationship. When discussing genital symptoms, people may describe "pain down there" or "discharge from the front" and may be uncomfortable using medically assigned terminology for anatomy. Follow-up questions to understand more specifically what is going on can mirror that person's language. For example, "When you say you are having discharge down there, do you mean it is coming from the front or the back? What kind of discharge is it?" or "When you say you are having pain in your lower region, is it on the inside or the outside?" Transmasculine people may use the term *front hole/genital canal* to describe the vagina.[9,19] In the text that follows, we have included an example of ways to approach various questions related to the sexual health and sexual practices of our patients.

SUPPORTING SEXUAL FUNCTION AND PLEASURE

Sexual pleasure derived during sexual activity is highly variable and personal. With this in mind, clinicians are always encouraged to ask questions that are (a) focused on obtaining clear information that will enhance or inform a physical exam; (b) introduced using some of the context questions; and (c) after being initiated, led by the patient in duration and focus. Stigma associated with pleasure from sexual activity can be a barrier for patient disclosure.[3] However, clinicians are encouraged to remain focused on the eliciting of relevant clinical information when asking questions specific to pleasure. We must be prepared to talk with our patients about sexual health behaviors, including but not limited to polyamory, use of sex toys, BDSM, and kink. See the text that follows for recommendations on how to engage with patients about how to use sex toys safely.

Safe Sex Toy Use

Sex toys can be used by all genders, alone or with pals and partners, and are a fun way of exploring new sensations and play. Sex toys come in different materials that require different types of upkeep to keep them body safe. There is no regulation in the sex toy industry and it is unknown whether ingredients may be toxic to consumers. However, clinicians can suggest patients give the toy a sniff for any heavy chemical smells and avoid buying toys from sex stores that do not have floor models that they can hold and analyze. Other sexual health-related communication practice recommendations can be found in the text that follows.[20]

COMMUNICATION ABOUT SEXUAL HEALTH

Starting Out

"As a component of your overall holistic healthcare, I have a few questions for you about your sexual health that I ask all of my patients."
　　"It is OK to not answer these questions today."
　　"I understand if some of these questions might feel uncomfortable. I am asking them so we can talk together about whether you might want to do any screenings or talk about ways to stay healthy."
　　"Do you have any specific concerns or questions we can start with, about your sexual health or sexual practices?"

Specific Practices

"How do you like to have sex?"
　　"What body parts go where when you are sexually active?"
　　"Are you physically intimate with more than one person?"
　　"Do you use condoms/barriers/dental dams/finger cots/etc.?"
　　"Do you currently exchange sex for money, housing, or food?"
　　"Do you experience any pain during or after sex?

(continued)

STI/HIV Information

"HIV is passed when bodily fluids from someone living with HIV come into contact with mucous membranes of your body (like your anus, vagina, or throat). Meaning there is not a barrier or condom to prevent the contact."

"Gonorrhea and chlamydia can be passed from person to person when there is contact from the tip of a penis to the throat, vagina, or anus; or when vaginal secretions come into close contact with the mucous membranes of a vagina, throat, or anus."

"Sharing sex toys can lead to passing HIV, gonorrhea, or chlamydia if they are not covered with a barrier or washed appropriately in between uses."

TRAUMA-INFORMED PHYSICAL EXAM

Conducting a trauma-informed physical exam requires adaptations and patient-centered decision-making. Several resources are available in the Supplemental Materials to guide clinicians on trauma-informed and pain-free speculum exams (Supplemental Materials are available on Springer Connect; visit connect .springerpub.com/content/book/978-0-8261-6921-1 and access the show supplementary dropdown). A physical exam of the genital and pelvic areas is extremely vulnerable, especially for people with previous sexual trauma and unsafe experiences in the healthcare system. About 15% of transgender people reported being asked invasive and inappropriate questions, often about their genitals or transgender status, during a medical encounter.[21] Previous negative and discriminatory experiences such as these contribute to a patient's hesitation to engage in any discussion or permission for physical contact from a provider.

When a thorough history and description of symptoms has been obtained, often times a modified physical exam may be sufficient, or the exam can even be deferred. The provider should always explain why a physical exam might help the clinician determine what is going on. But, the patient must be given the option to decline examination or only have part of the exam.

Self-collected swabs and self-speculum exams are also options to offer the patient. If the clinician suspects bacterial vaginosis or yeast, based on a history of white/yellow odorous pruritic vaginal discharge, but the patient has declined a pelvic exam, showing the patient how to obtain a self-collected swab of the discharge can provide adequate information to determine appropriate treatment.[22] The clinician could explain to the patient that conducting a simple external visual exam of the genitals may also provide more information, but that the internal speculum exam could be deferred. Alternatively, the clinician could collect the swab of the discharge, without needing to use a speculum, if the patient was uncomfortable doing self-collection. Additionally, providers may want to consider teaching people how to insert a vaginal speculum themselves, as it allows for a less uncomfortable experience. Patient education information about self-swabbing and self-speculum exams can be found at the links provided in the text box that follows.

- **Self-Swabbing Information**: www.feministmidwife.com/2012/09/27/self-swab/
- **How To Do A Cervical Self Exam**: www.womenshealthspecialists.org/self-help/cervical/
- **Self-Exam: The Cervix Close-Up**: www.ourbodiesourselves.org/book-excerpts/health-article/the-cervix-close-up/

CHRONIC PELVIC PAIN

Chronic pelvic pain is defined as any pelvic pain lasting longer than an arbitrary threshold of 6 months, and can be a challenging condition for individuals of any gender. As a part of the initial assessment of an individual's pain, it is essential to determine what the patient would consider an acceptable outcome of management.[19]

Comprehensive approaches to working up both chronic and acute pelvic pain have been noted in multiple publications.[19,23–25] There are numerous potential etiologies for pelvic pain, which may be comprised of any combination of physical, hormonal, and psychological sources. The International Pelvic Pain Society has a comprehensive *Pelvic Pain Assessment Form,* which is available on their website in English, French, Spanish, and Portuguese; the English version is gender neutral, though it does have some limitations that may need to be adapted, including the lack of specificity of types of sexual intercourse, the lack of a place to clarify a person's anatomy that is present or their gender identity, and a gendered drawing of an individual with breasts and hips which may be perceived to be a cis female.[26] Some potential causes of pelvic pain are as follows.

PELVIC PAIN ETIOLOGIES TO CONSIDER

Menstrual history (timing, frequency, even if amenorrhoeic)
Use of pain medication, association with testosterone dosing cycle
Sexual activity, pregnancy risk
STI/PID history
Surgical history: abdominal, laparoscopic, vaginal
Urinary symptoms
GI disturbance
Trauma history
Testosterone use (for transgender men)
Substance use

If imaging is indicated as a part of the workup, transabdominal, transvaginal, or trans-rectal ultrasound may all be considered based on the individual's anatomy present and their preferences for the method used.[19]

Effects of Testosterone:

- Cyclic pain related to testosterone dosing: Pelvic pain can be associated with testosterone administration, though the cause is undetermined. It can be treated with trauma-informed care, physical therapy, vaginal lubricants, or tricyclic antidepressants.[19] In one study, approximately one-fifth of individuals had a hysterectomy due to post-testosterone cramping, and another one-fifth due to cramping and bleeding.[27]
- Atrophy: Testosterone administration is associated with decreased estrogen in the vaginal tissue, which can result in thinning tissue, decreased elasticity, dryness, and friability. This can result in increased susceptibility to vaginitis and/or dyspareunia. Conservative treatments include vaginal lubricants and moisturizers. Vaginal estrogen may also be considered for comfort; it has limited systemic absorption and is not known to inhibit exogenous testosterone use.[19]

Concurrent mental health conditions: Association with gender incongruence or dysphoria may make pelvic exams more challenging for transgender individuals.[28] It has been well-established that chronic pelvic pain can be a comorbidity with mental health conditions such as posttraumatic stress disorder (PTSD) and depression.[25]

Trans men and ovarian cancer: Certain patients and providers may be concerned about increased risk of ovarian cancer for individuals who are taking testosterone. There have been isolated reports of ovarian cancer in trans men taking testosterone; however, there is no robust evidence that the risk is significantly higher for this population compared to cisgender women.[29] Several organizations state that there may be increased risk, which merits a risk-benefit discussion with patients, including the most recent *Standards* created by The World Professional Association for Transgender Health (WPATH), a guideline on transgender health published by The Endocrine Society, and a committee opinion on transgender health by the American College of Obstetricians and Gynecologists (ACOG).[30–32] The guidelines from The Center of Excellence for Transgender Health, by contrast, state that there is no increased risk for this population and that screening guidelines should be the same as they are for cisgender women.[33]

Hysterectomy and pain: Hysterectomy may be considered alongside other treatments of pelvic pain for individuals who may consider surgery, though it does not always relieve the pain.[19]

Vulvar pain: May use lidocaine 2% to 5% on cotton swab in vestibule, overnight for general pain, or 30 minutes prior to sexual activity.[19]

Pain management during vaginal procedures: May use topical lidocaine administered 10 minutes prior to the procedure, in combination with a low-dose benzodiazepine, such as 0.5 mg lorazepam, administered 30 minutes before the procedure.[19]

CONTRACEPTION, MENSES MANAGEMENT, AND ABORTION

Contraception for TGE Individuals

Contraception is needed for individuals of any gender who are at risk for unintended pregnancy.[34] This includes TGE individuals who have an intact uterus and are using testosterone. While testosterone may suppress menstruation, it does not reliably suppress ovulation and cannot be relied upon as contraception; there have been reported cases of TGE individuals on testosterone who have become unintentionally pregnant.[35] It is important for clinicians to appropriately counsel patients on this risk, as many individuals may still mistakenly believe that testosterone use will protect against pregnancy.[34,36]

There is no evidence that using estrogen-containing contraceptive methods while on testosterone will negatively impact the effects of the testosterone or present a safety risk.[37] Patients in need of contraception can be offered any contraceptive method that would be available to cis females.

Contraception for LGBQ Individuals

As a part of the sexual history taking, it is key to remember that an individual's sexual identity does not necessarily indicate the kinds of sexual behaviors they engage in. For example, a cis woman who identifies as a lesbian may also engage in sexual behaviors with individuals who have a penis. Furthermore, sexual fluidity appears to drive individuals' contraceptive decision-making.[38] The clinician should appropriately assess the risk for unintended pregnancy, and provide contraceptive counseling and care where indicated.[39] For individuals with a uterus, standard guidelines should be followed regarding the selection and initiation of a contraceptive method. For individuals with a uterus, currently the only contraceptive methods available in the United States are barrier methods and working with an individual's partner to use a Fertility Awareness Method (FAM).[40]

Contraception as Menses Management

For any individual who has unwanted or bothersome vaginal bleeding, hormonal contraceptive methods are first-line treatment.[41] Studies on the 52 mg LNG-IUD document a range of amenorrhea rates after 6 months of use from 15% to 54%; at the end of 2 years, amenorrhea rates range from 30% to 50%.[42,43] Rates of amenorrhea with DMPA appear to increase the longer this method is in use; research suggests that 25% of individuals experience amenorrhea at 6 months of DMPA use, and 46% to 75% at 12 months.[44,45] Information about menstrual suppression with testosterone therapy can be found in Chapter 9. Finally, emergency contraception is an option for all individuals who desire it, who may have had sex that could result in an unplanned pregnancy.

Abortion

As with all health services related to sexual and reproductive health, abortion care is accessed by individuals of all genders. Although there is limited research about the needs and preferences of TGE individuals who access abortions, available evidence suggests that barriers to abortion care are compounded for LGBTQIA+—and specifically, TGE—individuals.[46,47] Limited research suggests that unintended pregnancy is common for TGE individuals, including those using testosterone.[34,36] Abortion is needed for those who do not wish to continue their pregnancy.

To these authors' knowledge, there is no research about the type of abortion care that TGE individuals prefer, such as medication, clinic-based aspiration, or self-managed abortion. One trans "boy" shared in *Trans Bodies, Trans Selves* that when he elected to receive an in-office abortion procedure, he did so without revealing his gender: "A boy couldn't walk into this women's clinic. I felt I had no option but to become a woman for that two-hour stretch ... I was handed a light blue nightie with pink pigs all over it, and an over-washed flannel that looked like it should have belonged to a 70-year-old grandmother. Not something that I, as a boy with a baby, should be wearing."[48]

For individuals of all genders, medication abortion has been an increasingly common way to obtain an abortion in the United States; medication abortions accounted for just 6% of outpatient abortions shortly after the medication regimen was approved by the U.S. Food and Drug Administration (FDA) in 2000, and by 2014 this had grown to 31% of outpatient abortions.[49] Potential advantages of medication abortion is the possibility of increased privacy, and the possibility of avoiding a pelvic examination.[50]

Of particular note for NPs, PAs, and CNMs, legislation has been passed in several more states to allow non-physicians to provide abortions. Research supports the use of appropriately trained advanced practice clinicians (APCs) to provide safe early abortions.[51,52] Multiple national and international organizations support this as a means of expanding access to care, including the American College of Nurse Midwives, American College of Obstetricians and Gynecologists, American Public Health Association, and the International Confederation of Midwives.[53–56]

SAFER SEX: STI AND HIV PREVENTION AND TESTING

Safer sex means taking an approach to bacterial and viral sexually transmitted infection (STI) prevention that embraces multiple options and centers the patient experience in determining what is the best option for them.[57] For people who are engaging in sexual behaviors that involve contact with other bodies and bodily fluids, safer sex options can include specific prevention and testing mechanisms. Prevention methods include non-biomedical and biomedical approaches. Testing involves rapid result or send-out laboratory diagnostic testing.

Non-biomedical methods for preventing bacterial and viral STIs include barrier methods such as latex or non-latex condoms and dams. Patient education information about the various types of condoms and how to use them are available at www.plannedparenthood.org/learn/birth-control/condom. Condoms should be used with water-based lubricants; use of oil-based lubricants or Vaseline increase slippage and breaking of condoms.

Biomedical approaches to prevention involve HIV Pre-Exposure Prophylaxis (PrEP). PrEP involves taking a single tablet combination antiretroviral medication (tenofovir disoproxil and emtricitabine) once daily. Individuals who are at increased risk for HIV acquisition are candidates for PrEP. Any clinician can prescribe PrEP and guidelines for dosing and monitoring of PrEP therapy can be found at www.cdc.gov/hiv/guidelines/preventing.html.[58]

Testing for bacterial and viral STIs should be site-specific and routine, depending on the history of sexual behavior and timing of previous tests. Opt-out HIV testing is recommended at least once in a lifetime for all people between the ages of 13 and 64, or more frequently based on risk.[59] Testing for human papillomavirus (HPV) should be incorporated as per cervical cancer screening guidelines, and routine cervical cancer screening guidelines should be applied to all individuals with a cervix regardless of gender identity, expression, or sexual orientation. Transmasculine people on testosterone may have higher rates of inadequate cells on cytology. See Chapter 9 for more details about routine cancer screening in this population. Routine testing for herpes simplex virus is not recommended according to the 2015 CDC STI Screening Guidelines;[59] however, swab screenings are available for confirming diagnosis of genital ulcerative lesions. Gonorrhea and chlamydia are routinely found in the pharynx and anus, in addition to urethra and vagina. Screening should be site-specific and routine, depending on evaluation of risk. Self-collected anal swabs have been shown to be similarly sensitive to provider-collected swabs,[22] and they offer the advantage of patient autonomy, confidentiality and convenience.

CULTURAL SAFETY SUMMARY POINTS

- Clinicians should focus on building *partnerships* with LGBTQIA+ communities around sexual healthcare needs. Clinicians will need to employ verbal and nonverbal means of creating and building provider-patient trust, incorporating patient knowledge and experiences as vital components of the encounter.

- Clinicians can understand the *personal ADLs* of LGBTQIA+ patients when we utilize the 5 Ps of sexual history taking: Past STIs, Pregnancy plans and history, sexual Practices, sexual Partners, and Prevention of STIs/HIV.

- Practicing *purposeful self-reflection* allows the clinician to explore where we may be uncomfortable with sexual practices so we can expand our understanding in order to provide culturally safe care. Understanding our own blind spots will reduce implicit bias and expand our comfortability with discussing nontraditional sexual activities and lifestyles.

- Questions directed at patients should be relevant, contextualized, and appropriate within the scope of professional boundaries—allowing for *patient centering* where the clinician is focused on aligning the purpose of care with the patient's goals.

CONCLUSION

Sexual health is multifactorial and fluid despite overarching cultural narratives that promote cisgender-heteronormative-abelist ideals and hierarchies. Providers are responsible for recognizing diversity, honoring patient agency, and facilitating patient-directed goals. Clinicians can challenge dominant systematic exclusion and discrimination while creating new ways of centering patients during sexual health-focused visits.

REFERENCES

1. Centers for Disease Control and Prevention. Sexual health. Published June 25, 2019. https://www.cdc.gov/sexualhealth/Default.html

2. World Health Organization. Defining sexual health. Accessed January 23, 2020. http://www.who.int/reproductivehealth/topics/sexual_health/sh_definitions/en

3. Irvine JM. Sexualities: resisting sexual stigma for twenty years. *Sexualities*. 2018;21(8):1234–1237. doi:10.1177/1363460718772757

4. Herek GM. Beyond "homophobia": thinking about sexual prejudice and stigma in the twenty-first century. *Sex Res Soc Policy*. 2004;1(2):6–24. doi:10.1525/srsp.2004.1.2.6

5. Marsack J, Stephenson R. Sexuality-based stigma and depression among sexual minority individuals in rural United States. *J Gay Lesbian Ment Health*. 2017;21(1):51–63. doi:10.1080/19359705.2016.1233164

6. Goffman E. *Stigma: Notes on the Management of a Spoiled Identity*. Simon and Schuster; 1963.

7. Singer R. LGBTQ Training for obstetrical care providers in two urban settings: an examination of changes in knowledge, attitude and intended behavior. Published March 2016. https://search.proquest.com/openview/9951081849d694ffbbb8965e261dbe13/1?pq-origsite=gscholar&cbl=18750&diss=y

8. Phelan SM, Burgess DJ, Yeazel MW, et al. Impact of weight bias and stigma on quality of care and outcomes for patients with obesity. *Obes Rev.* 2015;16(4):319–326. doi:10.1111/obr.12266

9. Poteat T, German D, Kerrigan D. Managing uncertainty: a grounded theory of stigma in transgender health care encounters. *Soc Sci Med.* 2013;84:22–29. doi:10.1016/j.socscimed.2013.02.019

10. Minton HL. *Departing From Deviance: A History of Homosexual Rights and Emancipatory Science in America.* University of Chicago Press; 2002.

11. Gupta K. What does asexuality teach us about sexual disinterest? Recommendations for health professionals based on a qualitative study with asexually identified people. *J Sex Marital Ther.* 2017;43(1):1–14. doi:10.1080/0092623X.2015.1113593

12. Scherrer KS. Coming to an asexual identity: negotiating identity, negotiating desire. *Sexualities.* 2008;11(5):621–641. doi:10.1177/1363460708094269

13. Van Houdenhove E, Gijs L, T'Sjoen G, et al. Asexuality: a multidimensional approach. *J Sex Res.* 2015;52(6):669–678. doi:10.1080/00224499.2014.898015

14. Keuroghlian AS, Ard KL, Makadon HJ. Advancing health equity for lesbian, gay, bisexual and transgender (LGBT) people through sexual health education and LGBT-affirming health care environments. *Sex Health.* 2017;14(1):119. doi:10.1071/SH16145

15. DiNenno EA, Prejean J, Irwin K, et al. Recommendations for HIV screening of gay, bisexual, and other men who have sex with men—United States, 2017. *MMWR Morb Mortal Wkly Rep.* 2017;66:830–832. doi:10.15585/mmwr.mm6631a3

16. Maragh-Bass AC, Torain M, Adler R, et al. Risks, benefits, and importance of collecting sexual orientation and gender identity data in healthcare settings: a multi-method analysis of patient and provider perspectives. *LGBT Health.* 2017;4(2):141–152. doi:10.1089/lgbt.2016.0107

17. Speidel L, Jones M. *The Edge of Sex: Navigating a Sexually Confusing Culture From the Margins.* Routledge; 2019.

18. Nusbaum MRH, Hamilton CD. The proactive sexual health history. *Am Fam Physician.* 2002;66(9):1705–1712. https://www.aafp.org/afp/2002/1101/p1705.html

19. Obedin-Maliver J. Pelvic pain and persistent menses in transgender men. In: Deutsch MB, ed. *Guidelines for the Primary and Gender-Affirming Care of Transgender and Gender Nonbinary People.* Center of Excellence for Transgender Health, Department of Family and Community Medicine, University of California; 2016. https://transcare.ucsf.edu/trans?page=guidelines-pain-transmen

20. Brown University Health Promotion. What's the best way to clean sex toys? Accessed January 23, 2020. https://www.brown.edu/campus-life/health/services/promotion/content/whats-best-way-clean-sex-toys

21. James S, Herman J, Rankin S, et al. *The Report of the 2015 U.S. Transgender Survey.* National Center for Transgender Equality; 2016.

22. Ogale Y, Yeh PT, Kennedy CE, et al. Self-collection of samples as an additional approach to deliver testing services for sexually transmitted infections: a systematic review and meta-analysis. *BMJ Glob Health.* 2019;4(2):e001349. doi:10.1136/bmjgh-2018-001349

23. Kruszka PS, Kruszka SJ. Evaluation of acute pelvic pain in women. *Am Fam Physician.* 2010;82(2):141–147. https://www.aafp.org/afp/2010/0715/p141.html

24. Gasiewicz N, Romero M. Chronic pelvic pain. In: Likis FE, Schuiling KD, eds. *Women's Gynecologic Health.* 3rd ed. Jones & Bartlett Learning; 2017:711–770.

25. Speer LM, Mushkbar S, Erbele T. Chronic pelvic pain in women. *Am Fam Physician.* 2016;93(5):380–387. https://www.aafp.org/afp/2016/0301/p380.html

26. International Pelvic Pain Society. Documents & forms. Accessed June 15, 2019. https://www.pelvicpain.org/IPPS/Professional/Documents-Forms/IPPS/Content/Professional/Documents_and_Forms.aspx?hkey=2597ab99-df83-40ee-89cd-7bd384efed19

27. Rachlin K, Hansbury G, Pardo ST. Hysterectomy and oophorectomy experiences of female-to-male transgender individuals. *Int J Transgenderism*. 2010;12(3):155–166. doi:10.1080/15532739.2010.514220

28. Rachlin K, Green J, Lombardi E. Utilization of health care among female-to-male transgender individuals in the United States. *J Homosex*. 2008;54(3):243–258. doi:10.1080/00918360801982124

29. Harris M, Kondel L, Dorsen C. Pelvic pain in transgender men taking testosterone: assessing the risk of ovarian cancer. *Nurse Pract*. 2017;42(7):1–5. doi:10.1097/01.NPR.0000520423.83910.e2

30. World Professional Association for Transgender Health. Standards of care. Accessed February 19, 2019. https://www.wpath.org/publications/soc

31. Hembree WC, Cohen-Kettenis P, Delemarre-van de Waal HA, et al. Endocrine treatment of transsexual persons: an endocrine society clinical practice guideline. *J Clin Endocrinol Metab*. 2009;94(9):3132–3154. doi:10.1210/jc.2009-0345

32. American College of Obstetricians and Gynecologists. Committee opinion no. 512: health care for transgender individuals. December 2011. https://www.acog.org/clinical/clinical-guidance/committee-opinion/articles/2011/12/health care-for-transgender-individuals

33. Deutsch MB, ed. *Guidelines for the Primary and Gender-Affirming Care of Transgender and Gender Nonbinary People*. 2016. https://transcare.ucsf.edu/guidelines

34. Light A, Wang L, Zeymo A, et al. Family planning and contraception use in transgender men. *Contraception*. 2018;98(4):266–269. doi:10.1016/j.contraception.2018.06.006

35. Light AD, Obedin-Maliver J, Sevelius JM, et al. Transgender men who experienced pregnancy after female-to-male gender transitioning. *Obstet Gynecol*. 2014;124(6):1120–1127. doi:10.1097/AOG.0000000000000540

36. Abern L, Nippita S, Maguire K. Contraceptive use and abortion views among transgender and gender-nonconforming individuals assigned female at birth. *Contraception*. 2018;98(4):337. doi:10.1016/j.contraception.2018.07.027

37. Boudreau D, Mukerjee R. Contraception care for transmasculine individuals on testosterone therapy. *J Midwifery Womens Health*. 2019;64(4):395–402. doi:10.1111/jmwh.12962

38. Everett BG, Sanders JN, Myers K, et al. One in three: challenging heteronormative assumptions in family planning health centers. *Contraception*. 2018;98(4):270–274. doi:10.1016/j.contraception.2018.06.007

39. Charlton BM, Janiak E, Gaskins AJ, et al. Contraceptive use by women across different sexual orientation groups. *Contraception*. 2019;100(3):202–208. doi:10.1016/j.contraception.2019.05.002

40. Hatcher RA, Nelson A, Trussell J, et al. *Contraceptive Technology*. 21st ed. Ayer Company Publishers, Inc; 2018.

41. American College of Obstetricians and Gynecologists. Practice bulletin no. 136: management of abnormal uterine bleeding associated with ovulatory dysfunction. *Obstet Gynecol*. 2013;122(1):176–185. doi:10.1097/01.AOG.0000431815.52679.bb

42. Hidalgo M, Bahamondes L, Perrotti M, et al. Bleeding patterns and clinical performance of the levonorgestrel-releasing intrauterine system (Mirena) up to two years. *Contraception*. 2002;65(2):129–132. doi:10.1016/S0010-7824(01)00302-X

43. Bednarek PH, Jensen JT. Safety, efficacy and patient acceptability of the contraceptive and non-contraceptive uses of the LNG-IUS. *Int J Womens Health*. 2010;1:45–58. doi: 10.2147/ijwh.s4350

44. Hubacher D, Lopez L, Steiner MJ, et al. Menstrual pattern changes from levonorgestrel subdermal implants and DMPA: systematic review and evidence-based comparisons. *Contraception*. 2009;80(2):113–118. doi:10.1016/j.contraception.2009.02.008

45. Kaunitz A. Hormonal contraception for suppression of menstruation. *UpToDate*. Published September 2017. https://www.uptodate.com/contents/hormonal-contraception-for -suppression-of-menstruation

46. Fix L, Durden M, Obedin-Maliver J, et al. Perceptions regarding sexual and reproductive health care for transgender and gender-expansive people in the United States. Ibis Reproductive Health; 2018. https://ibisreproductivehealth.org/publications/perceptions -regarding-sexual-and-reproductive-health-carefor-transgender-and-gender

47. Hoffmann J, Bergin A. Contraception, abortion and more: understanding health disparities for LBGTQ patients in their own words [10G]. *Obstet Gynecol*. 2019;133:76S. doi:10.1097/01.AOG.0000558710.06533.3f

48. Hixson-Vulpe J. Preconceived notions. In: Erickson-Schroth L, ed. *Trans Bodies, Trans Selves: A Resource for the Transgender Community*. Oxford University Press; 2014:236. http://ebookcentral.proquest.com/lib/utah/detail.action?docID=1685668

49. Donovan M. Self-managed medication abortion: expanding the available options for U.S. abortion care. Guttmacher Institute. Published October 12, 2018. https://www .guttmacher.org/gpr/2018/10/self-managed-medication-abortion-expanding-available -options-us-abortion-care

50. American College of Obstetricians and Gynecologists. Practice bulletin no. 143: medical management of first-trimester abortion. *Obstet Gynecol*. 2014;123:676–692. doi:10.1097/01.AOG.0000444454.67279.7d

51. Weitz TA, Taylor D, Desai S, et al. Safety of aspiration abortion performed by nurse practitioners, certified nurse midwives, and physician assistants under a California legal waiver. *Am J Public Health*. 2013;103(3):454–461. doi:10.2105/AJPH.2012.301159

52. Patil E, Darney B, Orme-Evans K, et al. Aspiration abortion with immediate intrauterine device insertion: comparing outcomes of advanced practice clinicians and physicians. *J Midwifery Womens Health*. 2016;61(3):325–330. doi:10.1111/jmwh.12412

53. American College of Obstetricians and Gynecologists. Committee opinion number 613: increasing access to abortion. 2014. https://www.acog.org/clinical/clinical-guidance/ committee-opinion/articles/2014/11/increasing-access-to-abortion

54. American College of Nurse Midwives. Midwives as abortion providers. 2018. http://www .midwife.org/default.aspx?bid=59&cat=3&button=Search

55. International Confederation of Midwives. Essential competencies for midwifery practice. 2019. https://www.internationalmidwives.org/our-work/policy-and-practice/essential -competencies-for-midwifery-practice.html

56. American Public Health Association. Provision of abortion care by advanced practice nurses and physician assistants. Policy Number 20112. Published November 1, 2011. http://apha.org/policies-and-advocacy/public-health-policy-statements/policy-database/ 2014/07/28/16/00/provision-of-abortion-care-by-advanced-practice-nurses-and -physician-assistants

57. Crameri P, Barrett C, Latham J, et al. It is more than sex and clothes: culturally safe services for older lesbian, gay, bisexual, transgender and intersex people. *Australas J Ageing*. 2015;34:21–25. doi:10.1111/ajag.12270

58. Kamis KF, Marx GE, Scott KA, et al. Same-day HIV pre-exposure prophylaxis (PrEP) initiation during drop-in sexually transmitted diseases clinic appointments is a highly acceptable, feasible, and safe model that engages individuals at risk for HIV into PrEP care. *Open Forum Infect Dis.* 2019;6(7). doi:10.1093/ofid/ofz310

59. Workowski KA, Bolan GA. Sexually transmitted diseases treatment guidelines, 2015. *MMWR Recomm Rep Morb.* 2015;64(RR-03):1–137. https://www.cdc.gov/mmwr/preview/mmwrhtml/rr6403a1.htm

11

Perinatal Care for Trans, Gender Expansive, and LGBQIA+ Populations

Simon Adriane Ellis, Danielle Boudreau, Randi Singer, Ronni Getz, and Robin D'Aversa

LEARNING OBJECTIVES

By the end of this chapter, the reader will be able to:

- Identify barriers to achieving pregnancy and accessing pregnancy care for LGBTQIA+ individuals.
- Discuss how gender dysphoria may impact the transgender and gender expansive (TGE) patient experience of pregnancy and postpartum.
- Identify how to offer preconception counseling to LGBTQIA+ patients.
- Discuss best communication practices for the initial prenatal visit.
- Acknowledge the ways in which prenatal care of the TGE patient are similar to and different from prenatal care for the cisgender patient.
- Explain best communication practices during the labor and birth.
- Offer three ways that clinicians can modify their postpartum care to be LGBTQIA+ inclusive.
- Discuss three ways to support breast/chestfeeding for LGBTQIA+ parents.

INTRODUCTION

Though many LGBTQIA+ individuals desire children, and may wish to carry a pregnancy themselves, there is not clear information regarding the number of LGBTQIA+ individuals who have experienced pregnancy.[1] Limited research and ample anecdotal evidence, however, do support the fact that many LGBTQIA+ people can and do create families in a variety of ways, including through pregnancy. Understanding LGBTQIA+ experiences with fertility, pregnancy, and birth will allow clinicians to:

● Discuss fertility options before and after gender-affirming hormone therapy (GAHT).
● Discuss the roles of gender-affirming hormones on fecundity and potential birth outcomes.
● Support the physical and mental well-being of LGBTQIA+ individuals during pregnancy.

Overview

LGBTQIA+ people represent an underserved population. It is essential that TGE and other LGBTQIA+ individuals receive specific support during the perinatal period to address the psychological and emotional implications of conceiving, carrying a pregnancy, giving birth, and adapting to the postpartum period. Studies have found that the physical, hormonal, and social changes that are associated with the perinatal period can cause gender dysphoria, distress, and feelings of loneliness for TGE individuals.[1] Although studies are lacking, some research shows that the risk for unintended pregnancy among TGE individuals is approximately 25%.[2] Though this reported number of unintended pregnancies is half of what has been reported for cisgender populations, many TGE individuals have the added risk of potentially teratogenic exposure of testosterone to a developing fetus. Additionally, due to stigma and social rejection, TGE adolescents and young adults are disproportionately more likely to experience homelessness compared to their cisgender peers, increasing their exposure to health-related risks.[3-6] As many as 50% of TGE people have experienced intimate partner violence,[7] and 47% of TGE individuals report having experienced sexual assault at some point in their lifetime.[8] Finally, as has been previously discussed and what merits continued discussion, TGE individuals face significantly more barriers to accessing healthcare compared to the general population.[9,10]

Limitations to This Chapter

Broadly speaking, the majority of existing research regarding perinatal care does not assess the needs and experiences of LGBTQIA+ individuals. There are some exceptions to this rule, and these bodies of research will be cited throughout this chapter. While these studies are a start, in order to generalize about what may benefit an entire population of people, the sample sizes must be larger and the subjects more diverse. This dearth of data makes it challenging to create guidelines for an under-researched population.[11]

A Note on Intersecting Identities

As with all other aspects of sexual and reproductive healthcare, in perinatal care it is important to remember that patients' intersecting identities will shape their experiences as well as their health outcomes.[12-14] As has been discussed in Chapter 3, perinatal outcomes in the United States such as low birth weight babies, maternal and infant mortality, and rates of cesarean birth are worse for African American, American Indian, and Alaska Native women. (The bulk of this research examines outcomes for "women" without a discussion of gender.) Access to healthcare and a multitude of health markers—including insurance status, obesity, and psychological distress—are worse for individuals living in poverty.[6] Clinicians providing perinatal care to individuals of any gender must remember to practice the cultural safety and trauma-informed care frameworks that have been intentionally woven throughout this text.

BARRIERS TO ACCESSING PERINATAL CARE FOR LGBTQIA+ PATIENTS

LGBTQIA+ individuals face a multitude of barriers to accessing healthcare. It bears repeating that discrimination is detrimental to patient care.[4,15] LGBTQIA+ patients are not only subject to culturally unsafe care but may be denied healthcare altogether. Additionally, structural or legal factors further complicate the healthcare experience for LGBTQIA+ patients.[6,16] Unwieldy electronic health record (EHR) systems and insurance claims issues surrounding the discrepancy between a patient's sex assigned at birth, their legal sex, and their gender identity are a few of the common experiences which serve to support institutional discrimination and barriers to adequate care.[17] Consider, for example, how some EHR systems may only allow a new pregnancy episode to be opened for a female-designated patient. If the EHR lacks the flexibility to create a pregnancy episode for male and TGE patients, clinicians may end up documenting the visit in a way that misrepresents the patient's gender identity in order to proceed with the initial visit. This inaccurate documentation can negatively impact the patient's care and increase the likelihood of clinical staff mis-gendering the patient throughout their entire pregnancy (Case Study 11.1).

Case Study 11.1

Jon is a 32-year-old G2P0 at 8 weeks EGA by LMP equal to first trimester ultrasound. Jon and their husband, Mark, were very anxious about their first prenatal visit. In addition to the usual worries about the health of the pregnancy, they were both aware that Jon's insurance and medical record listed them as female and used their legal name. Jon was prepared at this initial visit to explain that their identity did not match the insurance information, and request that all staff and healthcare providers call then Jon and use masculine or they/them pronouns for them. The midwife, the nurse, and the billing person were receptive and affirming in their response that day by calling Jon by their correct name and using they/them pronouns as requested. When the couple left that first visit, they were relieved and felt seen. Jon and Mark returned for their 12-week visit excited to hear the heartbeat for the first time. They were sitting in an exam room waiting to be seen by the midwife. A nurse came in to assess vital signs and, noting two men in the room, stated, "Is she in the bathroom?" Jon's heart sank. Sitting there, with their urine cup in hand, they had to do it all again. Jon told the nurse about the insurance issue, that they are the pregnant one, that their name is Jon, and that they use masculine or they/them pronouns. The nurse quickly grabbed the chart on the door, made a notation, and apologized clumsily. This happened at nearly every visit, which affected Jon's prenatal and other care experience poorly.

Healthcare disparities are rooted in the lack of knowledge and discriminatory attitudes of healthcare providers; these often grow out of the cissexist, heteronormative assumptions that prevail as cultural norms. The most direct way to address barriers to healthcare experienced by sexual and gender minorities is through healthcare provider education.[18] The climate of perinatal care has been changing to include human reproduction for LGBTQIA+ families since the 1980s.[19] Perinatal healthcare providers must follow suit and demonstrate empathy and awareness of the discrepancy between those who have been supported in their reproductive goals (i.e., white, cisgender, heterosexual people) and those who have not.[20] Furthermore, because it is illegal to refuse assistive reproductive care to someone based on sexual orientation or gender identity, perinatal healthcare providers and fertility specialists are all required to care for those who identify as TGE.[21,22] As such, there is an urgent need for adequate education in providing perinatal care for TGE individuals.

A study by Light et al., focusing on transgender men's obstetrical care experiences,[23] reiterates the need for research into perinatal care for all TGE patients (of note, study participants include gender expansive individuals although the data is reported using the term *transgender men*). The main conclusion from this small study was that TGE people who want to reproduce are looking for healthcare providers who respect and understand them, and who are knowledgeable about their specific healthcare needs. This should be easily attainable. Patients want care providers who respect and understand them. End. Of. Story. In an earlier study by Grant et al., TGE patients were surveyed by the U.S. Department of Health to assess their particular healthcare experiences. TGE patients continue to report feeling marginalized by their healthcare providers.[4,5] In the 2015 follow up on the original Grant study, for example, 8% of those TGE people surveyed reported being denied gender-affirming care, 24% reported having to educate their healthcare provider about TGE health, and 33% of those surveyed reported at least one negative experience with a healthcare provider in the past year that they believed to be related to their gender identity.[24] The stigma associated with identifying oneself as TGE has been shown to correspond not only with intentional avoidance of seeking healthcare, but also with rates of suicide and suicidal attempts that are significantly higher than the national average.[4,25] What follows is just one example from *Trans Bodies, Trans Selves*, which illustrates how microaggressions expressed by a healthcare provider negatively affected one individual's willingness to seek future care.

> I avoid healthcare providers due to my gender identity. I experienced severe discrimination when I identified myself as queer in terms of sexual orientation, and I realize that gender is even less understood.[26]

This common response to avoid or delay healthcare makes sense given the maltreatment TGE communities have experienced by their healthcare providers.[16,24,25,27] For example, some TGE individuals report having been subject to unnecessarily long physical examinations because clinicians are curious about how they may or may not have altered their genitalia.[4] A clinician satisfying their own curiosity through a voyeuristic experience of a patient's examination is unethical, unacceptable, and in direct conflict with culturally safe patient care.

TGE individuals do reproduce, and they, like all childbearing patients, require knowledgeable support from medical professionals.[23] This chapter will focus on best perinatal clinical care practices for those whose sex assigned at birth was female but now identify as male, masculine of center, non-binary, or otherwise gender expansive. For the purpose of this book, perinatal care will include preconception through the postpartum period.

Gender Dysphoria During the Perinatal Period

Research has demonstrated that the perinatal period can be a time of increased dysphoria for many TGE individuals.[1,14,23] For TGE individuals specifically, gender dysphoria can be defined as marked emotional or psychological distress associated with the discrepancy between an individual's true gender and the sex that they were assigned at birth. The experience of dysphoria is unique to each individual, and may be fluid in response to a variety of physical, social, occupational, temporal, and psychological factors.

Powerful cultural narratives can create discomfort for anyone who is considering, experiencing, or recovering from the bearing of children; these narratives are overwhelmingly heteronormative and cisgendered.[28] TGE individuals who engage in family-building through pregnancy and birth struggle on a daily basis with strict cultural messages that associate childbearing with femininity. Being TGE and pregnant can mean risking being mis-gendered in public and clinical spaces. Research has shown that feelings of isolation can be common for TGE individuals in the prenatal and postpartum periods, which can compound experiences of dysphoria and other challenges to mental, emotional, and psychological well-being.[1]

The physical changes that occur during pregnancy may exacerbate some individuals' experience of dysphoria.[23,29] Growth in chest tissue, development of a "baby bump," and the cessation of gender-affirming hormone therapy (GAHT) can all be difficult for some TGE individuals. It may be challenging for some individuals to find gender-appropriate clothing that fits them during the later stages of pregnancy, or that conceals their chest tissue if they are choosing to do so. Some individuals may want to conceal their pregnancy, and some may not. The clinician should be assessing and affirming their patients' individual experiences and needs at all stages of the perinatal period.

Dysphoria may present in different ways and at different times; examples of these instances are pointed out throughout this chapter. Overall, the clinician should work to support the whole health of their patients by helping the patient to identify sources of support that are available to them during this transformative time.

Support for TGE Care From Professional Organizations

All perinatal care clinicians should anticipate that they will be called upon to provide perinatal care to TGE individuals. Different professional organizations have voiced varying levels of support for TGE-affirming care. Of particular note for perinatal care, the two most predominant midwifery organizations have had recent and public debates about TGE inclusive care. There is an ongoing debate and struggle within the American College of Nurse Midwifery (ACNM) about the delineation of TGE clinical care as a set of core competencies. TGE gender-affirming care—particularly care of transfeminine people—continues to be highly debated; at the time of this writing, discussions have not resolved.[30] American College of Obstetricians and Gynecologists (ACOG) posits that all OB/GYNs may provide preventive care for TGE people without any specialized training or consultation, but may need to refer out or consult before providing gender-affirming treatments.[31]

Preparing Your Practice to Provide Perinatal Care to TGE Individuals

In order to provide inclusive and culturally safe care, the clinical setting needs to be welcoming and affirming for peoples of all identities. By including images of diverse families on the walls of the clinic, by prominently displaying pronouns on your name-tag, or by wearing a rainbow pin on your lanyard or lab coat, you are communicating with your patient before you even open your mouth to speak. All staff should be trained in best practices for providing care specifically to TGE individuals, who are often left out of more generalized trainings on LGBTQIA+ care. Local TGE and LGBTQIA+ advocacy groups or public health offices are good resources to start with to find local training. A number of national organizations also have published online webinars and training materials; see Supplemental Materials for a full list of resources (Supplemental Materials are available on Springer Connect; visit connect.springerpub .com/content/book/978-0-8261-6921-1 and access the show supplementary dropdown).

As previously acknowledged, the physical space can be made to be inclusive through the thoughtful placement of posters and photographs that represent individuals of all genders and racial backgrounds, the inclusion of chairs in the waiting room which will fit all body types, and the placement of LGBTQIA+-inclusive visuals within each room. A clinic or hospital nondiscrimination policy should be made public and placed in visible locations in the healthcare setting, including the waiting room and check-in desks. Sample language for nondiscrimination policies can be found on the Human Rights Campaign website, or the ACLU website.[25,32,33] For example, the American Medical Association (AMA) recommends that a sign be hung in all clinical settings stating, "This office appreciates the diversity of human beings and does not discriminate based on race, age, religion, ability, marital status, sexual orientation, sex, or gender identity." If using an EHR, special attention needs to be paid to ensuring that patients' correct (even if not legal) name, pronouns, and gender are visible. Remember Jon? Having an EHR that prominently displays important gender identity information on the patient banner could have saved Jon and their partner much distress throughout the course of Jon's pregnancy. If using an EHR that does not have this capability, Jon's care team could have used fields such as the "nickname" field to prominently display their correct name and pronouns.

Administrative staff may also need to spend extra time ensuring insurance coverage for pregnancy-related services for patients, regardless of legal sex. Educational materials need to be edited to be gender-neutral and inclusive of all family and parenting structures. See Supplemental Materials for examples (visit connect.springerpub.com/ content/book/978-0-8261-6921-1 and access the show supplementary dropdown). A detailed discussion of creating a welcoming office environment is addressed in Chapter 4 on microaggressions and the aforementioned Supplemental Materials.

PRECONCEPTION AND CONCEPTION CARE

Preconception Counseling

While many individuals choose to see a care provider to discuss optimal preparation for pregnancy, not all individuals do. According to a study published in 2016, 45% of all U.S. pregnancies are unplanned,[34] and in a small qualitative study looking at the pregnancy experiences of 41 trans men, one-third of pregnancies were unplanned[23]; as such, preconception counseling should not be limited to one specific office visit for individuals of any gender. According to Lanik,[35] preconception counseling can take place at any office visit for a woman of childbearing age.

Like the majority of research related to pregnancy, Lanik[35] addresses the needs of heterosexual, cisgender women of childbearing age. For the purpose of this chapter, ACOG's 2017 position statement on preconception counseling[35] has been modified to be gender-inclusive. In order to reach individuals of all gender identities, preconception counseling should occur between the ages of 12 to 52 for all individuals whose sex assigned at birth was female.[2,31] Those whose sex assigned at birth was female may have nearly 40 years during which reproduction may occur. As such, it is imperative to acknowledge the possibility of pregnancy with all patients who may have the ability to reproduce. In order to minimize the potential for unfavorable perinatal outcomes for individuals with the capacity to reproduce, care providers must address the potential ramifications of intended and unintended pregnancy.

ACOG recommends that all care providers ask the following question of women of childbearing age: "Would you like to become pregnant within the next year?"[36] This question allows for individuals to share openly about their reproductive plans, concerns, and need for support and guidance. The authors of this text encourage healthcare providers to address the subject of pregnancy with all patients of childbearing age whose sex assigned at birth was female, not just those who identify as women. In a qualitative research study assessing the needs of TGE individuals who wished to start a family through becoming pregnant, a common theme was a lack of support by healthcare providers during the preconception period; the feeling of loneliness during the time prior to pregnancy was a pervasive finding among TGE individuals.[37] As such, healthcare providers must not only acknowledge that TGE patients may have the capacity to become pregnant, but they must also support TGE patients desiring pregnancy through affirming preconception support, as well as local and online resources that connect patients to other pregnant or postpartum patients.

Participants in the previously mentioned study encouraged providers to use a two-step approach for assessing reproductive plans. Step 1: Ask "Are you interested in becoming a parent (or having additional children) someday?" Step 2: If the patient answers affirmatively, following up with an open-ended question such as "Have you thought about how you would like to become a parent?" Unlike the pregnancy-specific question suggested by ACOG, these questions are not built on assumptions about how a person might want to build their family, and create space for greater exploration and acceptance of any route to parenthood the patient is considering.

PRECONCEPTION KEY QUESTIONS

1. Are you interested in becoming a parent (or having additional children) someday?
2. Have you thought about how you would like to become a parent (or have additional children)?

TGE Fertility

Like with all patients, understanding how to best support the fertility of TGE patients requires understanding of their medical history prior to preconception. Not all TGE people choose to undergo medical or surgical gender affirmation. For those who do, it is not certain how or if gender-affirming treatments could impact future fertility.[38] The most assured way to safeguard gametes for possible future fertility attempts is to undergo fertility preservation prior to initiation of gender-affirming care; however, assistive reproductive options are often expensive and not covered by insurance, a point that should be included in discussion with patients.[39,40]

Reassuringly, a recent study demonstrated no difference in outcomes of ovarian stimulation for assisted reproductive technology (ART) between cisgender women, TGE individuals who had not undergone gender-affirming testosterone therapy, and TGE individuals who had been on testosterone for up to 17 years.[41] This small study was limited to individuals seeking gamete retrieval for ART and the results cannot be generalized to all conception among TGE individuals assigned female at birth. However, the findings—coupled with ample anecdotal evidence of TGE conception after GAHT—offer hope that testosterone may not significantly impact long-term fertility.

It is important to note that at the moment of initiating gender-affirming care, the majority of transgender patients are of reproductive age[39]; as such, it is important that healthcare providers who facilitate medical or surgical gender affirmation inquire about the patients' family-building goals and be transparent about the fact that it is unknown if GAHT could have reproductive consequences.

Regarding gender-affirming genital/reproductive organ surgery, future reproductive options depend largely on which procedures are performed. Depending on the type of surgery, patients may be able to either become pregnant themselves or to contribute genetic material to a pregnancy gestated by another individual. Those who undergo metoidioplasty (release of the clitoral ligaments to create a phallus) without hysterectomy, for example, retain their full capacity to preserve gametes or to conceive and give birth. Pregnancy is not possible if the patient has had a hysterectomy. In the case of hysterectomy with oophorectomy, if gamete retrieval has not already been completed, genetic reproductive potential from the ovaries can possibly be retained through cryopreservation for subsequent insemination or in vitro fertilization using a gestational carrier such as the individual's partner or a surrogate.[38] Note that ovarian tissue cryopreservation is still experimental and may not be available or financially feasible for most patients.

Conception for TGE Individuals

As with all patients seeking to become pregnant, there are countless ways to bring an egg and sperm together. TGE individuals with ovaries, a vagina, and a uterus can become pregnant using sperm from a partner or donor who produces sperm. This can be done either via penetrative sex, intravaginal insemination (IVI), intracervical insemination (ICI), or intrauterine insemination (IUI). For some TGE patients who have partners who produce sperm, penis-in-vagina sex may not be a physically and/or emotionally comfortable method for insemination. Another option for establishing a pregnancy is to utilize previously cryopreserved oocytes or embryos. This is accomplished in combination with in vitro fertilization, either into the patient's own uterus or that of another gestational carrier, perhaps the patient's partner or a surrogate.[1] Considerations regarding method for insemination include personal preferences and experiences of dysphoria related to fertility methods, the reproductive capacity of the person with whom they are starting the pregnancy in the case of patients with partners or intended co-parents, financial barriers to fertility treatments or sperm banks, and many other factors.[9,23,38,39] The perinatal healthcare provider should discuss these options with TGE patients considering conception and, as with all patients, address individual medical and surgical history.

TESTOSTERONE KEY POINTS

- Testosterone = androgen replacement therapy as part of gender affirmation (gender-affirming hormone therapy [GAHT]).
- Major effects on ovarian function: usually leads to amenorrhea but ovulation can still occur; effects appear to be reversible even after prolonged use.
- Major effects on lactation: reduced milk production, due to unknown effects on nursing infant; patients are advised not to chestfeed if taking testosterone.
- Teratogenicity: testosterone is considered Pregnancy Category X based on limited and conflicting data. The primary concern regarding testosterone use during pregnancy is possible virilization of a female fetus. It is recommended that patients discontinue GAHT throughout the entire perinatal period, from attempting to conceive through the postpartum period for as long as chestfeeding continues.[23,42,43]
- Testosterone does not equal birth control. People at risk of becoming pregnant should use a form of birth control if they do not want to conceive.

Donor Versus Co-Parent

If an individual is using a known donor—meaning, a sperm donor who is personally known to them—it is important for all parties involved to set clear expectations up front. A sperm donor is not the same as a co-parent. If an individual is considering using a known donor without plans to co-parent the child, it is critical to undergo a legal process by which clear roles and boundaries are established. It is advisable for the individual who is seeking pregnancy to hire two attorneys: one for the gestational carrier, and one for the sperm donor. This will prevent future donor claims that a shared attorney was biased toward the interests of the intended parent(s).

CLINICAL PEARLS: CONCEPTION DECISIONS FOR TGE INDIVIDUALS

- *Whose sperm?* Partner versus sperm donor.
- *What type of sperm?* Fresh sperm versus frozen sperm, washed sperm versus non-washed sperm.
- *How will fertilization occur?* Penis-in-vagina intercourse versus insemination: intravaginal (IVI), intracervical (ICI), or intrauterine (IUI).
- *Is there a need for assistive reproductive technologies?* Physiologic pregnancy versus IVF/fertility treatments.
- *Who will carry the pregnancy?* The patient versus another gestational carrier such as a partner or surrogate.
- *What supports are available to the patient as they navigate their journey to parenthood?* Family, friends, medical providers, therapists, or peer support groups (online or in person).

A list of resources regarding fertility and conceptions that clinicians can give patients is included in the Supplemental Materials (Supplemental Materials are available on Springer Connect; visit connect.springerpub.com/content/book/978-0-8261-6921-1 and access the show supplementary dropdown).

Providing Insemination Services

Many clinicians may wish to include intracervical insemination (ICI) and intrauterine insemination (IUI) as a part of their practice. Of note, patients and sperm banks often use the term *ICI* interchangeably with *intravaginal insemination* (IVI) for insemination procedures performed without the assistance of medical professionals. Although technically different (insertion of sperm into the vaginal vault versus the endocervical canal), clinicians should be aware that patients may consider them the same procedure.

Although most research and writings regarding these insemination procedures focus on the needs and experiences of heterosexual, cisgender couples who are experiencing infertility, these are useful methods of achieving pregnancy for individuals who cannot or choose not to attempt conception via penis-in-vagina sex. IUI has historically been seen as the first-line approach to insemination, and limited data has found IUI to be more effective than ICI/IVI at achieving pregnancy in specific clinical scenarios, such as in the setting of unexplained infertility.[44] However, a 2018 Cochrane review found no clear benefit to IUI over ICI.[45] This review demonstrated no differences in live birth rates between IUI and ICI, regardless of whether cycles were stimulated by gonadotrophins.[46] Given that ICI is more cost effective than IUI and can be performed at home without any assistance from a medical professional, this method of insemination should be discussed with all patients considering insemination.

ICI and IUI are most often performed in outpatient clinic settings; however, some clinicians provide these services in clients' homes.[47] Those who have been marginalized and othered in clinical settings might choose the safety and support offered with an IUI at home.[48] Regardless of where it is performed, IUI is a sterile procedure that involves the insertion of prepared sperm into the uterus via a flexible catheter that is introduced through the cervical os. It should be performed at the time of predicted ovulation. It may be performed with or without superovulation that is stimulated by administration of medications and/or hormones.[49] The sperm sample should always be "washed" prior to IUI in order to minimize side effects and maximize chances of achieving conception. If a sperm sample has been procured from a sperm bank, it will typically already have been washed prior to being frozen and shipped to the patient.

Home IUI: A TGE Patient Perspective
When my partner and I were ready for me to try to get pregnant, we didn't want it to feel like a medical process. We just wanted it to feel like we were making a baby together. We were also worried about how we would be treated if we had insemination done in a clinic setting. We are both transgender/non-binary, and I had already had negative experiences at a fertility clinic. The fertility doctor was really focused on my gender identity and wouldn't spend much time talking about my actual concerns. He wasn't honest about what is really known and not known about pregnancy after being on testosterone for a long time, and he made inappropriate comments about how interesting/unique/odd it was that I wanted to get pregnant. I hated every second of our visits. The other staff at the clinic were nice to me, but I always felt really uncomfortable waiting in the lobby. I felt like the other patients were staring at me and I was always terrified that they would call me back from the lobby as "Mrs" or "Ms" because I'm marked as female in my chart. I didn't want to feel super stressed and on edge when my partner and I were making a baby. I didn't want to feel worried about being able to get onto the busy clinic schedule for an insemination visit at just the right time. And I didn't want to undergo a procedure performed by a stranger while I was laying naked in a cold room under a paper sheet. So my partner and I ended up working with a midwife from within our community, who has experience with home insemination. Scheduling was easy, there was no lobby to wait in, and I knew that no one was going to misgender myself or my partner during such an exciting, vulnerable, and scary moment for us. We got to be in our own warm, safe bedroom during the procedure, and our midwife did a great job of making sure my partner felt involved in the process. I felt so much love and gratitude toward both my partner and my midwife the whole time. I felt so good about the whole experience, I can't help but think that being so relaxed and happy contributed to us getting pregnant on the first try.

IUI and ICI procedures are within the scope of practice for nurse-practitioners, all midwives, and physician assistants with the appropriate training. For detailed training, online continuing medical education credits are available from the American Society for Reproductive Medicine on Assisted Reproductive Technologies and Procedures, and Semen Preparation for IUI (found at https://store.asrm.org/Learn/FindACourse.aspx as of the time of this writing).[50]

PRENATAL CARE

Introduction to Prenatal Care for TGE Individuals

Pregnancy can be an isolating or distressing experience, especially for TGE people.[23] Once pregnancy is achieved, the pregnant person then must attend frequent prenatal visits. As has been discussed, entering clinical spaces as a TGE person can be anxiety-provoking and may incur repeated instances of discrimination and marginalization.[51] Small studies published by Light et al. in 2014 and Ellis et al. in 2015 have shown that most TGE pregnant individuals have received prenatal and intrapartum care in hospital settings.[23,37] In both of these small studies, TGE individuals received midwifery care throughout pregnancy at higher rates compared to the general U.S. population: 18 out of 41 respondents in Light's study, and four out of eight respondents in Ellis's study, compared to 9.3% of the general U.S. population.[23,37,52] As a clinician, it is important to recognize the difficulties that may be involved for individuals who now will have monthly, biweekly, and weekly appointments. It is imperative to prepare clinical and hospital spaces to be comfortable and welcoming for people of all gender identities, which includes ensuring that all staff members are trained in TGE-inclusive care and communication.

Initial Prenatal Visit

The first prenatal visit sets the tone for an individual's prenatal care, regardless of gender identity. For TGE individuals, it is particularly important to establish cultural safety by confirming and using the individual's correct name and pronouns, validating their gender identity, and validating their family structure.[16,39,40] It is also an important time to discuss how they are feeling about being pregnant, and use reflective language to affirm their lived experience, which may or may not include new or increased feelings of gender dysphoria given the biological and social changes that pregnancy may bring. As with all patients who are newly pregnant, it is essential to determine whether or not this is a welcome pregnancy, and to provide full options counseling—including counseling on pregnancy termination—where warranted.[53] The remainder of this chapter will address caring for the patient who wishes to continue their pregnancy.

During the initial prenatal visit, a full history is taken which includes a personal medical history, social history, sexual history, family medical history, current and past medications, allergies, and past pregnancy history.[54] A full discussion of taking a sensitive sexual history is included in this book in Chapter 10 on sexual health. This visit is also typically the time when a physical exam and panel of prenatal labs are done, including some standard labs and some based on the individual's history[54,55]; recommended prenatal labs do not differ based on an individual's gender identity, and clinicians can follow general prenatal guidelines for this panel.

An initial OB physical exam should be performed with adaptations as needed. It is important to think critically about what exam components are truly necessary and to limit the exam to those components. For example, a pelvic exam is rarely necessary for a patient who has no current gynecologic concerns or symptoms and whose pregnancy dating will be based either on ultrasound or a certain LMP or insemination/IVF date.[56] For labs that may traditionally be gathered via pelvic examination, such as screening for gonorrhea and chlamydia, there are alternate options for specimen collection such as self-swabbing. Gonorrhea and chlamydia testing can also be completed using a urine test instead of a vaginal swab. When pelvic exams are indicated, self-speculum insertion can be offered. The details of these options are also included in the chapter on sexual health (Chapter 10).

Similarly, breast/chest exam is rarely necessary for a patient who has no current breast/chest concerns or symptoms; this is particularly true for patients who have undergone gender-affirming chest surgery. All proposed exam components should be discussed with the patient in advance of the exam and explicit consent should be obtained; patient autonomy should be honored when patients decline specific exam components or state a preference to wait for these to be performed until better rapport has been established. The entire physical exam can be deferred to a separate second appointment if this is helpful and no urgent concerns are present.

This initial prenatal visit is also a good time to discuss shared vocabulary for the person's body parts (i.e., what words do they use to refer to their genitalia and pelvic organs?) and to provide anticipatory guidance about the biologic and social changes associated with pregnancy, which may cause gender dysphoria, feelings of isolation, or discomfort for certain TGE individuals.[38] Clinicians should preemptively identify local options for behavioral health support, including TGE-knowledgeable counselors, and refer out frequently. Phone or online counseling may be a helpful option for patients living in areas without any local TGE-knowledgeable counselors. All clinicians in an office setting should be on the same page with referrals. As we would for "discomforts of pregnancy," utilize a handout that is current so that all clinicians are referring to the same vetted resources.

Routine Prenatal Visits

Following the initial prenatal visit, the schedule of prenatal care for TGE patients should be the same as for cisgender pregnant patients, although it may be helpful to have longer visit timeslots if possible. While pregnancies in TGE individuals are not inherently more medically complicated than in cisgender patients, they are different psychosocially. As such, clinician awareness and training related to a TGE patient's specific needs are essential in the culturally safe care of pregnant TGE patients. It should be recognized that there are unique psychosocial factors related to carrying a pregnancy when one does not identify as female; space should be created to discuss these concerns and provide support as desired by the specific patient. These areas of special consideration are highlighted at every visit in the sample schedule that follows. The authors of this text recommend that these psychosocial assessments be added to standard prenatal care when caring for TGE patients. Otherwise, clinicians should follow the prenatal care guidelines and schedules as established by their institutions; any deviations in clinical care should be based on clinical factors that arise.

Of note, it is important for the clinician to query themselves first when considering asking sensitive questions of their pregnant TGE patients: Is the intent of the question to satisfy one's own curiosity, or is it truly relevant to the patient's care? Creating space for discussion using compassion, empathy, and open-ended questions is appropriate, while asking irrelevant questions out of curiosity is inappropriate and constitutes a barrier to care.[9,10,27]

Sample Prenatal Visit Considerations

Early Pregnancy

TGE patients may reflect a wide range of responses to a new pregnancy. Some may feel relief to have conceived and now have a knowable time frame for how long they will have to experience the hormones of pregnancy, stay off testosterone, or wait to start testosterone for the first time. Whether or not they have undergone GAHT in the past, patients may begin to feel increased dysphoria in pregnancy, and/or they may also feel a new appreciation for their body's capacity to reproduce and create human life.

For patients who have undergone GAHT, clinicians should confirm that they have stopped taking testosterone. As should be done for all patients, screen for IPV, depression, suicidal thoughts or intentions, and drug/alcohol use—TGE individuals are at higher risk for all of these compared to the general population.[5,57] It is important to provide anticipatory guidance about the physiologic changes in pregnancy that may impact the individual's physical appearance. If they have recently stopped GAHT, now is a good time to review the phenotypic changes that are reversible with cessation of testosterone use: mainly, this includes the redistribution of body fat versus muscle mass, and the potential regrowth of chest tissue.[58] If the individual has had masculinizing chest reconstructive surgery, it is important to discuss the possibility that chest tissue will expand. A small study by MacDonald et al. also found that study participants who tried to use chest binding during pregnancy reported that it was too painful, and discontinued binding while they were pregnant.[14] Within this same study, two individuals who were status post masculinizing chest reconstructive surgery reported quick-onset mastitis in the postpartum period, even without chest binding.[14] As such, clinicians and patients should discuss these possibilities for individuals who have both had and not had chest surgery.

GENETIC AND CARRIER SCREENING: SPERM DONATION, EQUITY, AND INTERSECTIONALITY

Counseling on genetic and carrier screening has long been a staple of early pregnancy care, and the potential ramifications of screening often go unquestioned by clinicians. It must be noted that genetic screening is always elective. As such, all patient communication should acknowledge that screening is usually a personal/family decision versus a medical decision; as with all patients, TGE people may have a wide range of perspectives on screening. It is important to acknowledge that some ethicists, disability rights advocates, and people with disabilities argue that genetic screening serves a long-term goal of eradicating people with disabilities from society.[59-61] One possible way to frame the discussion with patients is as follows:

> Genetic screening, carrier screening, and screening for neural tube defects are optional tests that different individuals may choose to have done or not done for a variety of reasons. Some people choose to do some or all of the testing because they might want to prepare differently for a child who may be affected by one of these conditions, or because they might decide to end the pregnancy. Some people might choose to not do any of the testing because it wouldn't change anything about the decisions they make in this pregnancy, or because it would make them more anxious. Whatever you decide is best for you and your family, we are here to support you.

If an individual has used an established sperm bank, the sperm donors have likely already undergone carrier screening for heritable genetic conditions, including cystic fibrosis, as is recommended by the American Society for Reproductive Medicine (ASRM). If an individual is planning to use a sperm donor outside an established sperm bank, such as eliciting sperm donation from a friend or family member (known donor), ASRM recommends that the donor is tested for heritable diseases, including cystic fibrosis, as indicated by their genetic history.[62] It should be remembered that standard contraception and preconception counseling for heterosexual cisgender women does not include a universal recommendation to screen partners for heritable diseases before having unprotected intercourse.[63] As such, a recommendation that only LGBTQIA+/TGE/single people should be required to do so represents an undue financial and emotional burden.[9,64] Certainly, this screening should be available to all people if desired, but it should not be used as a barrier to care.

12 Weeks

Routine screening for IPV, depression, suicidality, and drug/alcohol use should be considered at all perinatal visits with TGE patients—clinicians should use their judgment as to whether clinical tools such as the Patient Health Questionnaire 9 (PHQ-9) or the Edinburgh Postnatal Depression Screen (EPDS) should be used at each visit, or if these formal tools should be interspersed with informal open-ended inquiry. As they near the second trimester, pregnant TGE individuals may be starting to notice bodily changes such as breast/chest growth or the beginnings of a "baby bump"; this could increase dysphoria in some individuals. Additionally, concerns may be starting to arise regarding pregnancy disclosure—patients may be beginning to struggle with whether they will be open about their pregnancy, or if they will try to be "stealth" by consistently concealing their pregnancy.

Of note, body habitus plays a significant role in how easy it is to conceal a pregnancy—those with a naturally larger body habitus may find it much easier to conceal a gravid abdomen than those with a naturally smaller body habitus. Discussions of weight gain throughout the course of pregnancy should be both evidence-based and body-positive (as with patients of any gender identity); the TGE patient's perceptions of how weight gain may contribute to their safety and comfort during pregnancy should also be explored if concerns are present. For example, some patients may desire a larger or smaller weight gain in order to affect others' perceptions of their gender identity throughout pregnancy—these concerns should be validated, and an earnest conversation about risks of inadequate or excessive weight gain in pregnancy should be initiated if indicated.

Along with making decisions about pregnancy openness or concealment, patients may be starting to consider what their family narrative will be in the future—will they be open about being a gestational parent in some contexts, all contexts, or no contexts? Concerns about how to navigate pregnancy at work or school may also be arising. Use of open-ended questions about well-being and any concerns the patient may be having will allow the patient to guide discussion. This is also a good time to remind patients about accessible support resources such as TGE-knowledgeable counselors and social media online peer support groups.

Clinical considerations at this visit include initiation of low-dose aspirin for those with risk factors for developing preterm preeclampsia. Current research supports initiation of low-dose (81 mg) aspirin at 12 weeks gestation for individuals at increased risk.[65,66] The agreed-upon risk factors from the American College of Obstetricians and Gynecologists (ACOG) and the U.S. Preventative Services Task Force (USPSTF) include high risk factors (e.g., prior history of preeclampsia, chronic hypertension, etc.) and moderate risk factors (e.g., nulliparity, body-mass index above 30, age over 35, first-degree relative with a history of preeclampsia, African American ethnicity). ACOG and the USPSTF recommend initiation of low-dose aspirin at 12 weeks for individuals with one high risk factor, or with two or more moderate risk factors.[66,67] Though not codified by ACOG or the USPSTF, there are studies that indicate preeclampsia risk may be higher when pregnancy is achieved with sperm that the gestational carrier has not been exposed to before, such as with sperm donation.[68–70]

16 Weeks

When discussing the anatomy scan, be aware of the language being used. Avoid the well-intentioned but misguided question, "Are you going to find out the gender?" As has been established previously, sex and gender are distinct and unrelated. Clinicians should be precise with language about sex versus gender, and be aware that parents of any gender may choose not to find out the sexual anatomy of their baby. Focusing on the health-related indications for performing the anatomy scan—including an assessment of the fetus's major anatomical structures, cervical length, and placental location—may assist in avoiding discussion of the fetal sex. Clinicians should avoid participating in the recently increased hype over "gender reveal parties," which have become common in popular media.

TGE patients may be fearful of how they will be treated during the anatomy scan, as they will need to interact with a new set of medical staff including ultrasound technologists and radiologists. For cervical length and placental location, providers may want to help their patients pre-think before the anatomy scan appointment if they (the patient) would like to accept or decline a transvaginal/internal US if indicated. It is helpful to discuss with patients what they do or do not want included in the radiology referral. For example, gender identity, name, and pronouns used can be included in the radiology referral in order to create a smoother patient experience. Example text for a patient who wants gender identity information included could be: "This patient is a pregnant transgender person who uses they/them or he/him pronouns. His name is listed in the medical record as Jennifer, but please make sure all staff refer to him as Jon." Patients should always be asked for explicit consent before including such information, as not all patients will want every clinician and staff member to be aware of their gender identity.

Patient concerns about safety, misgendering, and dysphoria are likely ongoing as the pregnancy continues. As noted earlier, TGE patients may experience new or increased dysphoria, or feel more peace in their body and its reproductive capacity. Space should be allowed for discussion of concerns if desired, and support resources offered as appropriate.

20 to 24 Weeks

Review of the fetal anatomy scan should be performed at this visit, using caution with language as outlined previously, and routine screening for IPV, depression, suicidality, and drug/alcohol use should continue. Clinicians should discuss gestational diabetes and anemia testing and provide anticipatory guidance on what the glucose tolerance test entails. As with the anatomy scan, discussion should be offered as to whether the patient would like gender identity information provided on the lab requisition form. If the lab at your facility includes rooms with curtains/dividers between patient spaces rather than private individual rooms, you can request that the lab make every effort to provide a fully private space so the patient can feel as comfortable as possible.

As body changes become more obvious, patients may struggle with finding clothing that fits their growing abdomen while still being reflective of their gender identity. Those who prefer to conceal their pregnancy may be starting to struggle with how to do this. Others may be open about their pregnancy and struggling with the responses they are receiving from family, friends, and peers. Patients who are non-binary, usually perceived as female, or have never undergone GAHT may start to experience increased misgendering—even from those who have been consistently supportive in the past—and/or may find misgendering even more difficult to tolerate than usual. Those who were usually perceived as male before becoming pregnant may newly begin to experience misgendering or may continue to be consistently perceived as male. Those who are perceived as male may not be seen as pregnant regardless of whether they want to be or not. Responses to this may vary—some may experience a sense of loneliness, sadness, or loss at this lack of public support for and recognition of the incredible experience they are undergoing; others may feel relief that they are able to get safely through their day being perceived as a non-pregnant man. Still others may experience a combination of both of these feelings. All TGE patients may be starting to think about what parental terms they might use for themselves, and this could be particularly distressing for people with expansive or non-binary gender identities. As at all visits, open-ended inquiry should be used to allow the patient to guide discussion.

24 to 28 Weeks

If gestational diabetes and anemia testing has not already been discussed, these tests should be reviewed at this time and options for stewardship of the lab referral reviewed as previously noted. Childbirth education classes should also be discussed at this visit. Most resources on childbirth preparation are focused on the experience of cisgender women and are heterocentric in content. There is a dire need for TGE-inclusive prenatal education materials. More LGBTQIA+ friendly childbirth education classes and resources are being created and offered online. These are generally easy to find through a basic internet search.

One option for TGE patients is to seek out individual childbirth education sessions; it may be most helpful to start by looking at local LGBTQIA+-friendly childbirth educators and checking to see if they are open to providing services in this alternate format. Individual childbirth educators may be willing to integrate content on infant care and lactation into these sessions if desired, so parents don't have to struggle separately with how to secure this information.

28 to 34 Weeks

Conversation about planned mode of birth and birth preferences should be initiated during this period, as well as discussion of the patient's plan for infant feeding after birth. According to one study, a higher proportion of TGE individuals who had used testosterone underwent cesarean birth compared with those who reported no testosterone use (36% compared with 19%, respectively). Although this finding was not statistically significant, of those who underwent a cesarean, 25% cited the indication as "elective."[71] These findings indicate that some patients may not be comfortable having a vaginal birth.

This may feel challenging to some clinicians, particularly given the clearly documented difference in outcomes and long-term risks between these modes of delivery. However, while the medical risks of surgical versus vaginal birth remain unchanged, it is important to understand that a cesarean should not be considered truly "elective" if gender dysphoria is a significant barrier to vaginal delivery. With that said, the clinician must discuss the increased risks to morbidity and mortality that are associated with this surgery while allowing for a full exploration of the patient's needs and honoring patient autonomy. ACOG recommends that, in the absence of other medical indications for early or cesarean birth, elective cesarean should only occur after 39 weeks gestation, with comprehensive review of the surgical risks as well as a discussion that the risks of placenta previa, placenta accreta, and hysterectomy will increase with any subsequent pregnancies.[72]

Discussion of infant feeding plan should also be sensitive to the specific needs and realities of the TGE patient. Just as for cisgender parents, there are multiple options for TGE parents in how they choose to feed their infant after birth. These include but are not limited to chest/breastfeeding; chestfeeding with formula, one's own milk, or donor milk using supplemental devices; pumping and bottle-feeding with one's own milk; bottle-feeding donor milk; and bottle-feeding formula. The feeding plan will vary based on an individual's preferences and resources, as well as whether or not they have undergone chest reconstruction.[1,23] The gestational parent may also be in a relationship with a partner who would like to chest/breastfeed as well. Those who have decided not to chestfeed due to gender dysphoria concerns or gender-affirming surgery may have a range of feelings about this from relief to grief to guilt, and these feelings, as well as the decision not to chestfeed, should be acknowledged and validated. Care should be taken not to shame patients who will not be feeding their babies human milk. A detailed overview of infant feeding options can be found in the "Postpartum Care" section of this chapter.

When discussing birth preferences and infant feeding, it is important to note that patients may feel significant fear about how they will be treated during birth (whether surgical or vaginal), what will happen in the event of unexpected transfer of care or change in delivery location (particularly for those planning a home or birth center birth), and so on. In the case of hospital birth, the clinician should work with the hospital in advance to create a plan for a smooth admission process, reducing the risk of misgendering throughout the hospital stay, and identifying advocates on the unit who can assist the patient as needed. It is advisable to involve social work in this planning process. In the case of home birth or birth center birth, clinicians should help the patient explore in advance what hospital they would go to in the case of intrapartum transfer, and work with that hospital to create a plan. In all situations, the patient's needs, goals, and preferences should guide the planning process; what an ideal plan looks like may vary widely from patient to patient.

35 to 40 Weeks

As at all visits, screening for IPV, depression, suicidality, and drug/alcohol use should be performed. GBS screening should be discussed and performed, and the patient should be offered the option of self-swabbing if desired. Many clinicians offer a cervical sweep to individuals past 39 weeks gestation. This is a low-risk intervention that has been shown to decrease the chances of post-dates pregnancy.[73] Special consideration should be given to TGE individuals—as well as survivors of sexual trauma—prior to any digital pelvic exam. Visual or physical examination of the genitals may be the source of significant dysphoria for some TGE people, while others may not experience this.[29,74] This should be discussed in advance, and the clinician should elicit feedback from the patient as to what strategies might lessen the impact of dysphoria. It is also important to counsel patients on the sensations they can expect during cervical exam and possible cervical sweep.

Steps that clinicians can consider taking in order to provide culturally safe cervical exams include but are not limited to the following:

- Describe each step of the exam prior to its occurrence.
- Stand to the side of the individual's body, as opposed to in between their bent legs.
- Stand at the side of the table or bed, as opposed to sitting on the edge alongside the patient.
- Use all of the other steps outlined for providing a trauma-informed pelvic exam in Chapter 10.[75]

Regardless of whether cervical sweep will be performed, clinicians should discuss with all patients what cervical exams are and what they feel like, and indications for these exams. Patients should be reminded that their consent will be obtained before each examination and it is their right to decline any physical exam. A script of how to provide sensitive cervical exams, authored by Stephanie Tillman, CNM,[76] is included in the Supplemental Materials (Supplemental Materials are available on Springer Connect; visit connect.springerpub.com/content/book/978-0-8261-6921-1 and access the show supplementary dropdown). Labor support and pain management options should be discussed with all individuals who are electing to proceed with vaginal birth. Further discussion of this care is included in the "Intrapartum Care" section of this chapter.

INTRAPARTUM CARE

The intrapartum period can be an exciting time, when your patient is about to meet their baby for the first time. Depending on the practice setting, clinicians may or may not have had the opportunity to meet their laboring patient prior to the intrapartum period.

Language

The clinician should find out how the patient and their support person(s) would like to be addressed. Even if the clinician has cared for the patient throughout the prenatal period, it is important to confirm the patient's correct name and pronouns at the start of the intrapartum care. It is also important to confirm the name (or nickname) and/or pronouns the patient is using to refer to their baby, whether or not they know the anatomical sex of the fetus. Other terminology the clinician should be aware of includes how the patient is describing their own role and the role of their partner(s); individuals often use words such as *dad*, *carrier*, or *gestational parent* to affirm their gender identity and describe their parenting role; others may choose to use *mom* or similar terms—it is critical that the clinician not make assumptions about what the patient will prefer, or discount the difficulty they may experience making decisions about this. Additional language to confirm involves the words a patient uses to refer to their own anatomy. The clinician can say: "Everyone uses different words to describe their anatomy and I want to make sure I'm using the correct language when I take care of you today—could you tell me what words you use for your chest and genitals?" This responsive, professional, and time/situation bound question allows providers to follow patients' lead on language. People can refer to their body parts however they choose. As healthcare providers, it is our job to meet them where they are and reaffirm their identity through shared language. By meeting the patient with shared language, we acknowledge their reality as shared truth. This patient-centered language should be used in all aspects of intrapartum care, from discussion of labor physiology to walking the patient through steps of a laceration repair should it be necessary.

Throughout labor care, clinicians should be aware of the language that is used to talk about general epidemiology. For example, saying "most women experience spotting up to 6 weeks after birth" would not be patient-centered language if the patient in front of you does not identify as female. A good general practice is to start with gender-neutral language (i.e., "many new parents") and then move to individually affirming, patient-centered language once the patient's specific preferences are known (i.e., "many new dads"). The clinician should take the time to ensure that the other labor and birth staff members are willing and able to provide TGE-inclusive care. This may mean the clinician needs to advocate for use of the correct name, pronouns, and other terminology involved in respectful care of their patient. The clinician may also need to advocate for their patient with family members who may be present for the birth.

Examples of language the clinician can use to gather information is as follows:

- Hi, I'm _____ and I'll be the midwife taking care of you. I use _____ pronouns. What name do you go by? What pronouns do you use?
- And who are your support people with you today?
- Your baby is looking/sounding great on monitoring. Do they have a name that's public yet? (If not: Okay, how do you refer to your baby?)
- Everyone uses different words to describe their anatomy and I want to make sure I'm using the correct language when I take care of you today—could you tell me what words you use for your chest and genitals?

A Note on Cervical Exams

Cervical exams can be a useful part of intrapartum care. Providing comfortable cervical exams is important for patients of all gender identities, including TGE individuals. Utilizing trauma-informed care when performing cervical exams is always essential regardless of gender identity. But, because TGE patients often experience dysphoria in regard to their genitals, and are more likely to experience sexual violence than their cisgender counterparts, it is especially important with this patient population to utilize trauma-informed care during pelvic examinations.[39,64,74] As previously stated, the book's Supplemental Materials provide guidance on providing sensitive and comfortable cervical exams[77] (Supplemental Materials are available on Springer Connect; visit connect.springerpub.com/content/book/978-0-8261-6921-1 and access the show supplementary dropdown).

Training Birth Unit Staff in TGE-Affirming Care

There are numerous resources for training healthcare staff in how to provide TGE-affirming care. Clinicians should investigate local or regional resources for in-person or web-based training, and ensure that staff who fill a variety of roles in the healthcare setting—not just clinicians—attend these trainings. The National LGBT Health Institute created a short, 25-page guide for healthcare staff on providing inclusive care to LGBTQIA+ individuals, which can be useful in educating hospital staff.[78] In 2016 Lambda Legal updated a resource on implementing transgender-affirming hospital policies, including sample language for policies on respectful staff interactions with TGE patients, access to personal items that support an individual's gender presentation, and more.[33] Different clinical settings will find unique strategies to keep all staff well-informed about best practices. It may be useful to build a framework using the guiding principles of team-based care as outlined in a report generated by the ACOG Task Force on Collaborative Practice, including: place the patient at the center, involve the patient as a part of the team, create a shared team vision, clarify group roles, emphasize accountability, prioritize communication, and recognize that team leadership is "situational and dynamic."[79] Additional resources on TGE-affirmative best practices are available in Chapter 9 and the associated Supplemental Materials (Supplemental Materials are available on Springer Connect; visit connect. springerpub.com/content/book/978-0-8261-6921-1 and access the show supplementary dropdown).

Other ways clinicians can create a culturally safe, inclusive environment in the birthing room include:

- Wear a rainbow or LGBTQIA+-inclusive pin/sticker on hospital scrubs/badge/lanyard.
- When the baby is born, be mindful of not assigning a gender to the baby based on genitalia. Prior to the birth, clinicians should be sure to discuss with any other clinical staff who will be present that they should under no circumstances announce the baby's sex based on the anatomy that they see, unless that is the explicit stated desire of the parent/family.

POSTPARTUM CARE

As with the previous sections in this chapter, most aspects of postpartum care for TGE individuals are medically the same as care for individuals of any gender identity, but care should be tailored to meet the specific psychosocial needs of this population. Included in the text that follows are topics of special consideration for TGE patients in the postpartum period. Any time a clinician is meeting a family for the first time, it is important to confirm the names and pronouns of the parent as well as the infant.

ANTICIPATORY GUIDANCE FOR THE POSTPARTUM PERIOD

It is helpful to begin the conversation about aspects of the postpartum period during pregnancy. These topics include but are not limited to: subsequent pregnancy spacing or prevention, mental health and postpartum mood disturbance/depression, starting or resuming GAHT, and the social and legal implications of family building as a TGE individual.

- If the patient will be at risk for unintended pregnancy following the birth of their child, they will need contraception. A detailed discussion of pregnancy prevention for TGE individuals is included in Chapter 10.
- TGE individuals are at increased risk for mental health disorders compared to the general population;[20,38] this puts them at higher risk for postpartum depression. Start the conversation about identifying supports that the individual can make use of in the postpartum period; these include but are not limited to social supports such as meal trains and chore sharing, behavioral health counseling, pharmacologic mood stabilization, yoga, meditation, diet, and other lifestyle changes that can optimize postpartum mood adjustment.
- Discuss possible desire to start or resume testosterone after giving birth. Further discussion is included in this section.
- In addition to the typical array of fears and anxieties that all parents face as they approach the end of their pregnancies, TGE patients may be grappling even more intensely at this point with what their family narrative will be, what parental terms they plan to use, and how their family, friends, and peers will respond to them as parents. Some patients may feel fear that their parental rights could be challenged by members of their or their partner's families of origin who are not supportive of their gender identity; many TGE people are aware of both recent and historical examples of parents losing custody of their children due to the perception that being TGE makes them an unfit parent. Creating space for discussion of any fears and offering support and validation may be especially helpful during the heightened vulnerability of late pregnancy. Referrals for mental health, peer support, or legal resources should be offered as appropriate.

Infant Feeding After Chest Masculinization and GAHT

As is true for all patients, a TGE person's decision about how to feed their newborn is a personal one. Healthcare providers should discuss pertinent risks and benefits of all infant feeding options and support each patient in the informed choice that is best for them and their family. It is possible for some TGE patients with a history of testosterone use and/or chest masculinization surgery to nurse their infant; we will discuss specifics of this in the text that follows.

INSTEAD OF SAYING *BREAST* **OR** *BREASTFEEDING,* **TRY ...**

- Chest, chestfeeding
- Nursing
- Lactation
- Infant feeding

To begin with, let us consider the language most commonly used to describe nursing: "breastfeeding." As discussed earlier in this chapter, some people in the TGE community use different terms to refer to their body parts. In the context of infant feeding, one such example is to substitute "chest" for "breast," which may feel more comfortable for TGE patients. Clinicians should avoid the word *breast* when discussing infant feeding until they know how the patient refers to this process; instead, use gender-neutral words like *chest* and *chestfeeding, nursing, lactation,* and *infant feeding.*[77] As discussed previously, clinicians should always check in with the patient about the words they prefer to use to talk about their body.

If an individual has undergone any medical or surgical gender-affirming interventions, it may change aspects of their infant feeding plan. Each situation is considered in turn in the text that follows.

Surgical Chest Reconstruction

Some patients may have undergone masculinizing chest reconstructive surgery prior to conception; see Chapter 9 on surgical gender-affirming procedures for an overview. While chestfeeding may be possible after certain forms of chest reconstruction, the impact of chest masculinization surgery is not always predictable.[1,14] There are two primary factors that would impact future chestfeeding ability: amount of remaining ductal mammary tissue and nipple patency (in the case of surgeries where nipple grafting is completed). Even if trying to preserve chestfeeding ability by tailoring surgical technique, results will always be unpredictable and there is no way to guarantee chestfeeding potential. We know this to be true in cisgender women who undergo breast surgery as well.

As part of an informed consent process, surgeons who perform this type of surgery should discuss with their patients the potential impacts on lactation prior to surgery.[38] With this information, some patients may choose to defer chest reconstruction until after the completion of childbearing if they strongly desire to chestfeed.[1] As discussed earlier, some individuals are able to chestfeed successfully after surgery; others may experience mastitis or engorgement without ability to remove milk from the chest due to a lack of nipple patency—should these occur, standard treatment regimens (lactation suppression measures, antibiotic therapy, etc.) should be utilized.

Chest-Binding Postpartum

The decision about if and when to use chest-binding in the postpartum period is also not well studied. There is at least one published report of an individual who gradually resumed chest-binding when his infant was 10 months old, without reported complications.[14]

Gender-Affirming Hormone Therapy

History of GAHT use does not preclude individuals from being able to chestfeed. If chestfeeding or pumping with bottle feeding is desired, it is recommended to do so without concurrent testosterone use.[80,81] This recommendation exists in order to support both successful lactation as well as infant safety. Elevated testosterone levels have been shown to suppress lactation, which could lead to insufficient milk production.[80] The effects of testosterone on a chestfed infant are unknown.[38] From limited data, testosterone does not appear to pass into milk in significant levels or have any short-term impact on infants.[81] As is true about most lactation recommendations, without substantial evidence proving lack of associated harm, the recommendation at this time remains to avoid concurrent testosterone use while nursing. If a patient does resume or initiate testosterone while nursing, they should be advised to do so under the care of the child's pediatrician, who may counsel them on recognizing signs of androgen exposure in the infant.[38]

In the postpartum period, the decision to chestfeed may coincide with the decision about when to start or resume testosterone if desired. A study of 41 TGE individuals who experienced pregnancy after transition found that those who had a history of testosterone use were less likely to chestfeed than those who had not previously used testosterone.[23] Healthcare providers should be attuned to their TGE patients' unique experience of gender dysphoria that may accompany the postpartum period; both the continued lack of GAHT during chestfeeding as well as the social perception of nursing as a traditionally feminine role can be sources for dysphoria. All individuals who choose not to chestfeed should receive standard counseling on lactation suppression techniques, with language tailored to the specific needs of the individual.

Alternatives to Chestfeeding

Alternatives to chestfeeding are the same for TGE people as they are for cisgender people. At the most basic level, formula and donor milk are options. Some non-gestational partners may choose to induce lactation themselves. The most common method of lactation induction is the Newman-Goldfarb protocol, which involves a combination of combined oral contraceptives, breast massage, pumping, domperidone, and herbal support. The full protocol can be found at www.canad ianbreastfeedingfoundation.org/induced/regular_protocol.shtml. Transfeminine individuals can also modify this protocol in order to induce lactation—the primary modification involves adjusting doses of feminizing GAHT, with addition and titration of micronized progesterone if not already included in the individual's GAHT regimen, rather than using combined oral contraceptives.[82,83]

Regardless of the method of infant feeding, the known benefits of bonding can still be achieved through many alternative feeding practices. A supplemental nursing system (SNS) can help facilitate bonding between the infant and one or more parents. These devices consist of a container for holding milk or formula and an attached tube, the end of which is placed alongside the nipple. When the infant latches to the nipple and begins to suckle, milk is transferred from the holding container into the infant's mouth. This nursing system is suitable both as the sole source of milk, or as a supplement to a low milk supply in the chest for any reason, including status post chest reconstruction.[14] Alternative feeding systems are used not only by TGE parents[83,84], but also by adoptive parents, parents through surrogacy, and other non-gestational parents.[85] SNS devices can be purchased through a broad array of online and brick-and-mortar establishments, including Amazon, Target, and directly from the Medela breast pump company, and range in cost from approximately $18 to $60 as of the time of this writing.

Postpartum Depression

Rates of suicide and depression are higher among TGE individuals than their cisgender counterparts.[50,86] One qualitative study of transgender men who experienced pregnancy suggests that this population may be at an increased risk for postpartum depression.[23] In that same study, many participants noted common feelings of isolation and loneliness throughout pregnancy, and cited a lack of TGE-sensitive resources for postpartum depression. The authors of that study recommend an emphasis on the assessment of peripartum mood changes in the TGE population. The first page of the Edinburgh Postnatal Depression Scale (EPDS) is gender-neutral, and can be printed as a single-side only tool for assessment of postpartum depressive symptoms—see Supplemental Materials (Supplemental Materials are available on Springer Connect; visit connect.springerpub.com/content/book/978-0-8261-6921-1 and access the show supplementary dropdown). The authors of this chapter recommend leaving off the second page, which is intended as scoring instructions for clinical providers, and references "mothers." A 2013 ACOG committee opinion on postpartum care recommends contact with a care provider within the first 3 weeks postpartum, rather than waiting until the common 6-week visit.[87]

As has been discussed previously in this chapter, clinicians can help individuals identify strategies for combating loneliness and isolation during the perinatal period, including identifying both new and existing sources of support. These support systems may include inherited or chosen family, friends, faith communities, neighbors, work colleagues, and online communities. Strategies identified in the previous section on Anticipatory Guidance for the Postpartum Period included the mobilization of a support network to assist with a meal train or chore sharing, and the utilization of behavioral health or complementary health services such as counseling, yoga, acupuncture, meditation, massage, or any other stress management techniques. After the baby is born, the clinician should help the patient revisit whatever plan for postpartum well-being was established; if a plan was not previously established, it is not too late to do so. Pharmacologic support may also be considered on a case-by-case basis.

Resuming or Starting Androgen Therapy

As has been discussed throughout this chapter, the cessation of GAHT is recommended throughout the entire perinatal period: from the time the patient begins attempting to conceive through the postpartum period, as long as chestfeeding continues. For some individuals, this time period may feel like a very long time to be off of testosterone. No recommendations exist regarding ideal timing for starting or resuming GAHT after birth. As such, it can be a collaborative decision between patient and clinician made on a case-by-case basis. Considerations include the individual's desired infant feeding method, and a discussion of the lack of evidence regarding GAHT use during lactation.[81] Some clinicians may be concerned about a theoretical risk of VTE with taking testosterone during the hypercoagulable state of the early postpartum period; however, this risk is likely quite minimal, particularly with titration of testosterone dose over time and routine monitoring of hematocrit and hemoglobin. As an example to support this approach, testosterone is generally not discontinued for other common hypercoagulable states such as after surgery, and lab monitoring is not required. Based on self- and provider assessment, the risks and benefits to the individual's mental, emotional, physical, and social well-being should be considered, especially in decisions to postpone GAHT.[38] The risk of depression and suicidality with delayed starting or resumption of gender-affirming hormone therapy should be included in this risk/benefit analysis.

Postpartum Contraception

Discussions about an individual's care in the postpartum period should include an assessment of their future pregnancy intentions, and risk for unintended pregnancy. If an individual is planning to resume GAHT, it is important to remind them that testosterone may not fully prevent ovulation and thus is not an effective contraception method.[58] Individuals of any gender identity have been shown to experience unplanned pregnancy, including in TGE populations.[23,41,88] Although the research is limited regarding contraception for TGE individuals, including those who are taking testosterone, all currently available contraceptive methods appear to be safe and reasonable for use within this population.[88] There is no research that indicates a difference in the timing of postpartum contraception initiation for cisgender versus TGE individuals. A more robust discussion of contraception considerations for TGE individuals is included in Chapter 10.

Pelvic Floor Dysfunction and Therapy

Particular attention must be given to the pelvic floor of postpartum LGBTQIA+ patients. Those who identify as TGE may experience increased dysphoria with pelvic floor dysfunction and required therapy. As such, pelvic floor therapy referrals must be made only to those whose practice aligns with the cultural safety of LGBTQIA+ patients.[42]

CULTURAL SAFETY SUMMARY POINTS

- Some but not all TGE people experience dysphoria, which can be expressed as a feeling of deep unease or conflict, in regard to their bodies—particularly in regard to the more socially gendered body parts such as the breasts/chest, genitals, and reproductive organs.[29,74]
- Gender affirmation is not linear or standardized; instead, it is a deeply nuanced and personal process, and individuals' needs and desires may change over time. Not all TGE people seek medical or surgical gender-affirming care.[58,89,90]
- Some but not all TGE people lack support from or connection with their families of origin; this may limit their financial and emotional support resources during pregnancy and parenting.[91]
- Current discrimination and historical trauma impact TGE individuals' willingness to seek medical care, as well as their comfort with seeking medical care.[4,15]
- Not all TGE pregnant people will come out to their provider as TGE—some people who have expansive or non-binary gender identities may be perceived as female, and choose to "fly under the radar" with their care providers to avoid discrimination. This can increase feelings of isolation and distress.[15,16,27]
- Language matters! Using gender neutral language with ALL patients will create an environment in which TGE individuals may feel more comfortable disclosing their gender identity. Providers should make a practice of starting with gender neutral language and then moving toward gender-affirming language as defined by the individual patient.[16,26,58]

CONCLUSION

Perinatal care for TGE individuals is an area of healthcare in need of much more research and attention. The medical care of TGE individuals from preconception to the postpartum period has sometimes subtle and sometimes deep differences which demand our most loving attention. Clinicians can best support TGE individuals during the perinatal period if they make a conscious effort to listen to and affirm the unique experience of each of their patients.

REFERENCES

1. Obedin-Maliver J, Makadon HJ. Transgender men and pregnancy. *Obstet Med.* 2016;9(1):4–8. doi:10.1177/1753495X15612658
2. Francis A, Jasani S, Bachmann G. Contraceptive challenges and the transgender individual. *Womens Midlife Health.* 2018;4(12). doi:10.1186/s40695-018-0042-1
3. Herek GM. Beyond "Homophobia": thinking about sexual prejudice and stigma in the twenty-first century. *Sex Res Soc Policy.* 2004;1(2):6–24. doi:10.1525/srsp.2004.1.2.6
4. Grant J, Mottet L, Tannis J. *Injustice at Every Turn: A Report of the National Transgender Discrimination Survey.* National Center for Transgender Equality; 2011. https://www.transequality.org/sites/default/files/docs/resources/NTDS_Report.pdf
5. Institute of Medicine (U.S.), ed. *The Health of Lesbian, Gay, Bisexual, and Transgender People: Building a Foundation for Better Understanding.* National Academies Press; 2011.
6. Lim FA, Brown DV, Justin Kim SM. Addressing health care disparities in the lesbian, gay, bisexual, and transgender population. *Am J Nurs.* 2014;114(6):24–34. doi:10.1097/01.NAJ.0000450423.89759.36
7. Stiles-Shields C, Carroll RA. Same-sex domestic violence: prevalence, unique aspects, and clinical implications. *J Sex Marital Ther.* 2015;41(6):636–648. doi:10.1080/00926 23X.2014.958792
8. Smith SG, Zhang X, Basile KC, et al. *The National Intimate Partner and Sexual Violence Survey (NISVS): 2015 Data Brief—Updated Release.* National Center for Injury Prevention and Control, Centers for Disease Control and Prevention; 2018.
9. Berger AP, Potter EM, Shutters CM, Imborek KL. Pregnant transmen and barriers to high quality healthcare. *Proc Obstet Gynecol.* 2015;5(2):1–12. doi:10.17077/2154-4751.1285
10. Roberts TK, Fantz CR. Barriers to quality health care for the transgender population. *Clin Biochem.* 2014;47(10–11):983–987. doi:10.1016/j.clinbiochem.2014.02.009
11. Makadon HJ. Ending LGBT invisibility in health care: the first step in ensuring equitable care. *Cleve Clin J Med.* 2011;78(4):220–224. doi:10.3949/ccjm.78gr.10006
12. Bertrand M, Kamenica E, Pan J. Gender identity and relative income within households. *Q J Econ.* 2015;130(2):571–614. doi:10.1093/qje/qjv001
13. Crenshaw K. Mapping the margins: intersectionality, identity politics, and violence against women of color. *Stanford Law Rev.* 1991;43(6):1241. doi:10.2307/1229039
14. MacDonald T, Noel-Weiss J, West D, et al. Transmasculine individuals' experiences with lactation, chestfeeding, and gender identity: a qualitative study. *BMC Pregnancy Childbirth.* 2016;16:106. doi:10.1186/s12884-016-0907-y
15. Cruz TM. Assessing access to care for transgender and gender nonconforming people: a consideration of diversity in combating discrimination. *Soc Sci Med.* 2014;110:65–73. doi:10.1016/j.socscimed.2014.03.032
16. Singer RB, Crane B, Lemay EP, et al. Improving the knowledge, attitudes, and behavioral intentions of perinatal care providers toward childbearing individuals identifying as LGBTQ: a quasi-experimental study. *J Contin Educ Nurs.* 2019;50(7):303–312. doi:10.3928/00220124-20190612-05
17. Callahan EJ, Sitkin N, Ton H, et al. Introducing sexual orientation and gender identity into the electronic health record: one academic health center's experience. *Acad Med.* 2015;90(2):154–160. doi:10.1097/ACM.0000000000000467
18. Sekoni AO, Gale NK, Manga-Atangana B, et al. The effects of educational curricula and training on LGBT-specific health issues for healthcare students and professionals: a mixed-method systematic review. *J Int AIDS Soc.* 2017;20(1):21624. doi:10.7448/IAS.20.1.21624

19. Blake V. It's an ART not a science: state-mandated insurance coverage of assisted reproductive technologies and legal implications for gay and unmarried persons. *Minn J Law Sci Technol.* 2011;12(2):651–715. https://scholarship.law.umn.edu/cgi/viewcontent .cgi?article=1145&context=mjlst

20. Ethics Committee of American Society for Reproductive Medicine. Access to fertility treatment by gays, lesbians, and unmarried persons: a committee opinion. *Fertil Steril.* 2013;100(6):1524–1527. doi:10.1016/j.fertnstert.2013.08.042

21. American Society of Reproductive Medicine. Counseling issues to discuss with gay men and lesbians seeking assisted reproductive technologies (ART). 2012. https:// www.reproductivefacts.org/news-and-publications/patient-fact-sheets-and-booklets/ documents/fact-sheets-and-info-booklets/counseling-issues-for-gay-men-and-lesbians -seeking-assisted-reproductive-technologies-art

22. American College of Nurse-Midwives. Position statement: transgender/transsexual/ gender variant health care. 2012. http://www.midwife.org/acnm/files/ACNMLibraryData/ UPLOADFILENAME/000000000278/Transgender%20Gender%20Variant%20 Position%20Statement%20December%202012.pdf

23. Light AD, Obedin-Maliver J, Sevelius JM, et al. Transgender men who experienced pregnancy after female-to-male gender transitioning. *Obstet Gynecol.* 2014;124(6):1120–1127. doi:10.1097/AOG.0000000000000540

24. James S, Herman JL, Rankin S, et al. *The Report of the 2015 U.S. Transgender Survey.* National Center for Transgender Equality; 2015.

25. Wichinski KA. Providing culturally proficient care for transgender patients. *Nursing.* 2015;45(2):58–63. doi:10.1097/01.NURSE.0000456370.79660.f8

26. Erickson-Schroth L, ed. *Trans Bodies, Trans Selves: A Resource for the Transgender Community.* Oxford University Press; 2014.

27. Singer RB. LGBTQ training for obstetrical care providers in two urban settings: an examination of changes in knowledge, attitude and intended behavior. March 2016. https://search.proquest.com/openview/9951081849d694ffbbb8965e261dbe13/1?pq-origs ite=gscholar&cbl=18750&diss=y

28. Singer RB. Improving prenatal care for pregnant lesbians. *ProQuest.* Accessed September 17, 2019. https://search-proquest-com.proxy.cc.uic.edu/docview/1095482667?accountid =14552&pq-origsite=summon

29. American Psychiatric Association. What is gender dysphoria? Accessed September 14, 2019. https://www.psychiatry.org/patients-families/gender-dysphoria/what-is-gender -dysphoria

30. Midwives Alliance of North America. Core competencies. Published July 12, 2012. https:// mana.org/resources/core-competencies

31. American College of Obstetricians and Gynecologists. Committee opinion no. 512: health care for transgender individuals. December 2011. https://www.acog .org/clinical/clinical-guidance/committee-opinion/articles/2011/12/health-care-for -transgender-individuals

32. Human Rights Campaign. Patient non-discrimination sample policies & statements. Accessed September 17, 2019. https://www.thehrcfoundation.org/professional-resources/ patient-non-discrimination

33. Lambda Legal. Creating equal access to quality health care for transgender patients: transgender-affirming hospital policies. Human Rights Campaign International, Hogan Lovells, New York City Bar. 2016. https://www.lambdalegal.org/publications/ fs_transgender-affirming-hospital-policies

34. Finer LB, Zolna MR. Declines in unintended pregnancy in the United States, 2008–2011. *N Engl J Med.* 2016;374(9):843–852. doi:10.1056/NEJMsa1506575

35. Lanik AD. Preconception counseling. *Prim Care.* 2012;39(1):1–16. doi:10.1016/j.pop.2011.11.001

36. ACOG. Prepregnancy counseling. 2019. https://www.acog.org/clinical/clinical-guidance/committee-opinion/articles/2019/01/prepregnancy-counseling

37. Ellis SA, Wojnar DM, Pettinato M. Conception, pregnancy, and birth experiences of male and gender variant gestational parents: it's how we could have a family. *J Midwifery Womens Health.* 2015;60(1):62–69. doi:10.1111/jmwh.12213

38. Hoffkling A, Obedin-Maliver J, Sevelius J. From erasure to opportunity: a qualitative study of the experiences of transgender men around pregnancy and recommendations for providers. *BMC Pregnancy Childbirth.* 2017;17(suppl 2):332. doi:10.1186/s12884-017-1491-5

39. T'Sjoen G, Van Caenegem E, Wierckx K. Transgenderism and reproduction. *Curr Opin Endocrinol Diabetes Obes.* 2013;20(6):575–579. doi:10.1097/01.med.0000436184.42554.b7

40. Amato P. Fertility options for transgender persons. In: Deutsch MB, ed. *Guidelines for the Primary and Gender-Affirming Care of Transgender and Gender Nonbinary People.* 2nd ed. Center of Excellence for Transgender Health, Department of Family and Community Medicine, University of California San Francisco; 2016:100–102. www.transhealth.ucsf.edu/guidelines

41. Leung A, Sakkas D, Pang S, et al. Assisted reproductive technology outcomes in female-to-male transgender patients compared with cisgender patients: a new frontier in reproductive medicine. *Fertil Steril.* 2019;112(5):858–865. doi:10.1016/j.fertnstert.2019.07.014

42. Light A, Wang L, Zeymo A, et al. Family planning and contraception use in transgender men. *Contraception.* 2018;98(4):266–269. doi:10.1016/j.contraception.2018.06.006

43. Light A, Stark B, Gomez-Lobo V. Fertility, pregnancy, and chest feeding in transgendered individuals. In: Kovacs CS, Deal CL, eds. *Maternal-Fetal and Neonatal Endocrinology.* Elsevier; 2020:505–513. doi:10.1016/B978-0-12-814823-5.00028-3

44. Carroll N, Palmer JR. A comparison of intrauterine versus intracervical insemination in fertile single women. *Fertil Steril.* 2001;75(4):656–660. doi:10.1016/s0015-0282(00)01782-9

45. Kop PA, Mochtar MH, O'Brien PA, et al. Intrauterine insemination versus intracervical insemination in donor sperm treatment. *Cochrane Database Syst Rev.* 2018;(1). doi:10.1002/14651858.CD000317.pub4

46. O'Brien P, Vandekerckhove P. Intra-uterine versus cervical insemination of donor sperm for subfertility. In: The Cochrane Collaboration, ed. *Cochrane Database of Systematic Reviews.* John Wiley & Sons, Ltd; 1998. doi:10.1002/14651858.CD000317

47. Keenan J. Beyond the turkey baster. *Slate.* Published August 26, 2013. https://slate.com/human-interest/2013/08/intrauterine-insemination-at-home-midwives-are-performing-iuis-without-formal-education-or-regulation.html

48. Mamo L. Negotiating conception: lesbians' hybrid-technological practices. *Sci Technol Hum Values.* 2007;32(3):369–393. doi:10.1177/0162243906298355

49. Hoffman BL, Schorge JO, Bradshaw KD, et al. Treatment of the infertile couple. In: Schorge JO, Hoffman BL, Schaffer JI, et al. eds. *Williams Gynecology.* 3rd ed. McGraw Hill Professional; 2016:449–470.

50. American Society for Reproductive Medicine. Find a course. Accessed March 20, 2019. https://store.asrm.org/Learn/FindACourse.aspx

51. National Center for Transgender Equality. National Transgender Discrimination Survey. Accessed February 19, 2019. https://transequality.org/issues/national-transgender-discrimination-survey

52. Martin JA, Hamilton BE, Osterman MJK. *Births: Final Data for 2015*. National Center for Health Statistics; 2017.

53. Moss DA, Snyder MJ, Lu L. Options for women with unintended pregnancy. *Am Fam Physician*. 2015;91(8):544–549. https://www.aafp.org/afp/2015/0415/p544.html

54. King TL, Brucker MC, Fahey J, et al. *Varney's Midwifery*. 5th ed. Jones & Bartlett Learning; 2015.

55. Zolotor AJ, Carlough MC. Update on prenatal care. *Am Fam Physician*. 2014;89(3): 199–208. https://www.aafp.org/afp/2014/0201/p199.html

56. National Collaborating Centre for Women's and Children's Health (UK). *Clinical Examination of Pregnant Women*. RCOG Press; 2008. https://www.ncbi.nlm.nih.gov/books/NBK51890

57. Beal J. Bridget Lee Fuller: Mayflower myth vs. historic midwife. *Midwifery Today Int Midwife*. 2015;(115):50–52. https://midwiferytoday.com/mt-magazine/issue-115

58. Deutsch MB, ed. *Guidelines for the Primary and Gender-Affirming Care of Transgender and Gender Nonbinary People*. Center of Excellence for Transgender Health, Department of Family and Community Medicine, University of California San Francisco; 2016. www.transhealth.ucsf.edu/guidelines

59. Hansen I. Promoting a more inclusive understanding of sexual assault and interpersonal violence. *J Sex Med*. 2017;14(5 suppl 4):e288. doi:10.1016/j.jsxm.2017.04.363

60. Miller PS, Levine RL. Avoiding genetic genocide: understanding good intentions and eugenics in the complex dialogue between the medical and disability communities. *Genet Med*. 2013;15(2):95–102. doi:10.1038/gim.2012.102

61. Gillott J, Screening for disability: a eugenic pursuit? *J Med Ethics*. 2001;27(suppl 2):ii21–ii23. doi:10.1136/jme.27.suppl_2.ii21

62. Thomas GM, Rothman BK. Keeping the backdoor to eugenics ajar?: disability and the future of prenatal screening. *AMA J Ethics*. 2016;18(4):406–415. doi:10.1001/journalofethics.2016.18.4.stas1-1604

63. Boudreau D, Mukerjee R. Contraception care for transmasculine individuals on testosterone therapy. *J Midwifery Womens Health*. April 2019. doi:10.1111/jmwh.12962

64. The Practice Committee of the American Society for Reproductive Medicine and the Practice Committee of the Society for Assisted Reproductive Technology. Recommendations for gamete and embryo donation: a committee opinion. *Fertil Steril*. 2013;99(1):47–62.e1. doi:10.1016/j.fertnstert.2012.09.037

65. Safer JD, Coleman E, Feldman J, et al. Barriers to health care for transgender individuals. *Curr Opin Endocrinol Diabetes Obes*. 2016;23(2):168–171. doi:10.1097/MED.0000000000000227

66. Roberge S, Bujold E, Nicolaides KH. Aspirin for the prevention of preterm and term preeclampsia: systematic review and metaanalysis. *Am J Obstet Gynecol*. 2018;218(3): 287–293.e1. doi:10.1016/j.ajog.2017.11.561

67. Rolnik DL, Wright D, Poon LC, et al. Aspirin versus placebo in pregnancies at high risk for preterm preeclampsia. *N Engl J Med*. 2017;377(7):613–622. doi:10.1056/NEJMoa1704559

68. U.S. Preventive Services Task Force. Final recommendation statement: low-dose aspirin use for the prevention of morbidity and mortality from preeclampsia: preventive medication. 2014. https://www.uspreventiveservicestaskforce.org/Page/Document/RecommendationStatementFinal/low-dose-aspirin-use-for-the-prevention-of-morbidity-and-mortality-from-preeclampsia-preventive-medication

69. Kyrou D, Kolibianakis EM, Devroey P, et al. Is the use of donor sperm associated with a higher incidence of preeclampsia in women who achieve pregnancy after intrauterine insemination? *Fertil Steril.* 2010;93(4):1124–1127. doi:10.1016/j.fertnstert.2008.12.021

70. Smith GN, Walker M, Tessier JL, Millar KG. Increased incidence of preeclampsia in women conceiving by intrauterine insemination with donor versus partner sperm for treatment of primary infertility. *Am J Obstet Gynecol.* 1997;177(2):455–458. doi:10.1016/s0002-9378(97)70215-1

71. González-Comadran M, Urresta Avila J, Saavedra Tascón A, et al. The impact of donor insemination on the risk of preeclampsia: a systematic review and meta-analysis. *Eur J Obstet Gynecol Reprod Biol.* 2014;182:160–166. doi:10.1016/j.ejogrb.2014.09.022

72. Mylonas I, Friese K. Indications for and risks of elective Cesarean section. *Dtsch Ärztebl Int.* 2015;112(29-30):489–495. doi:10.3238/arztebl.2015.0489

73. American College of Obstetricians and Gynecologists. Cesarean delivery on maternal request. 2019. https://www.acog.org/clinical/clinical-guidance/committee-opinion/articles/2019/01/cesarean-delivery-on-maternal-request

74. American Psychiatric Association. What is gender dysphoria? 2013. https://www.psychiatry.org/patients-families/gender-dysphoria/what-is-gender-dysphoria

75. Boulvain M, Stan C, Irion O. Membrane sweeping for induction of labour. *Cochrane Database Syst Rev.* 2005;2005(1):CD000451. doi:10.1002/14651858.CD000451.pub2

76. Tillman S. Feminist midwife scripts: painful cervical exams during labor. *Feminist Midwife.* http://www.feministmidwife.com/2016/04/04/feminist-midwife-scripts-painful-cervical-exams-during-labor/#.X7BNQlNKi8o

77. Jennings J, Nielsen P, Buck ML, et al. Collaboration in practice: implementing team-based care: report of the American College of Obstetricians and Gynecologists' Task Force on Collaborative Practice. *Obstet Gynecol.* 2016;127(3):612–617. doi:10.1097/AOG.0000000000001304

78. Kabiri D, Hants Y, Yarkoni TR, et al. Antepartum membrane stripping in GBS carriers, is it safe? (The STRIP-G study). *PLoS One.* 2015;10(12):e0145905. doi:10.1371/journal.pone.0145905

79. National LGBTQIA+ Health Education Center. *Providing Inclusive Services and Care for LGBT People: A Guide for Health Care Staff.* The Fenway Institute; 2016. https://www.lgbthealtheducation.org/publication/learning-guide

80. Wolfe-Roubatis E, Spatz DL. Transgender men and lactation: what nurses need to know. *MCN Am J Matern Nurs.* 2015;40(1):32–38. doi:10.1097/NMC.0000000000000097

81. Gorton R, Buth J, Spade D. *Medical Therapy and Health Maintenance for Transgender Men: A Guide For Health Care Providers.* Lyon-Martin Women's Health Services; 2005.

82. LactMed. Testosterone. *Drugs and Lactation Database.* October 19, 2020. https://www.ncbi.nlm.nih.gov/books/NBK501721/

83. Reisman T, Goldstein Z. Case report: induced lactation in a transgender woman. *Transgender Health.* 2018;3(1):24–26. doi:10.1089/trgh.2017.0044

84. Glaser RL, Newman M, Parsons M, Zava D, Glaser-Garbrick D. Safety of maternal testosterone therapy during breast feeding. *Int J Pharm Compd.* 2009;Jul-Aug;13(4):314–317. PMID: 23966521.

85. O'Kane C. Photos of "breast-feeding" dad go viral. *CBS News.* July 3, 2018. Accessed March 3, 2020. https://www.cbsnews.com/news/photos-of-breastfeeding-dad-go-viral

86. Witcomb GL, Bouman WP, Claes L, et al. Levels of depression in transgender people and its predictors: results of a large matched control study with transgender people accessing clinical services. *J Affect Disord.* 2018;235:308–315. doi:10.1016/j.jad.2018.02.051

87. American College of Obstetricians and Gynecologists. Committee opinion no. 736: optimizing postpartum care. *Obstet Gynecol.* 2018;131:e140–e150. doi:10.1097/AOG.0000000000002633

88. Cipres D, Seidman D, Cloniger C, et al. Contraceptive use and pregnancy intentions among transgender men presenting to a clinic for sex workers and their families in San Francisco. *Contraception.* 2017;95(2):186–189. doi:10.1016/j.contraception.2016.09.005

89. Reisner SL, Bradford J, Hopwood R, et al. Comprehensive transgender healthcare: the gender affirming clinical and public health model of fenway health. *J Urban Health.* 2015;92(3):584–592. doi:10.1007/s11524-015-9947-2

90. Stroumsa D, Shires DA, Richardson CR, et al. Transphobia rather than education predicts provider knowledge of transgender health care. *Med Educ.* 2019;53(4):398–407. doi:10.1111/medu.13796

91. Seibel BL, de Brito Silva B, Fontanari AMV, et al. The impact of the parental support on risk factors in the process of gender affirmation of transgender and gender diverse people. *Front Psychol.* 2018;9:399. doi:10.3389/fpsyg.2018.00399

Afterword: A Call to Action

Ronica Mukerjee, Randi Singer, Linda Wesp,
and Pia Pauline Lenon

As we write this conclusion, it is July of 2020 and our world as we knew it is both exactly the same and entirely different from when we began writing this book several years ago. The systems we work within continue to be shaped by intersecting systems of oppression. Voices rising against these systems are louder, but dismantling of the systems still needs to happen on every level.

Our biggest disappointment, now more than ever, would be that clinicians will read this text, close the book, and continue their usual method of care without initiating new actions to increase social justice for their patients. We are worried that you, our colleagues, will ask for more learning opportunities, more reading groups, and more continuing education, but that you won't do the necessary personal work to transform yourselves. That work, in conjunction with outward positive action, is exactly what is required, and although it should have started a long time ago, starting immediately will do. With privilege that comes from being in healthcare leadership roles comes the ability to forget and/or to simplify solutions. It is easier for us as faculty, staff, and students to say, "We understand the problems," but then shrug our shoulders and say that the system is too difficult to change. We implore you to remain uncomfortable.

Employ your knowledge of the five tenets of cultural safety: partnerships, personal activities of daily living (ADLs), prevention of harm, patient centering, and purposeful self-reflection (see Chapter 1). Utilizing this framework, providers will shift the power balance to patients through learning, through engaging in the struggle for body and community autonomy, through challenging police aggression and other biased violence, and through putting our brains and intellects and selves on the line too as much as is needed to create real, conscientious, and relevant change.

If this book has made a lasting impression on you, you will find yourself asking more complex questions than you will have simple answers. How do we turn an oppressive system into an opportunity for change? How do we restructure culturally and medically negligent healthcare systems into ones that reflect appropriate care for the most excluded people in healthcare? Patients who identify as part of the LGBTQIA+ population, particularly BIPOC (black, indigenous, people of color) people, experience a multitude of barriers to obtaining healthcare, and many of these barriers stem from providers' lack of knowledge regarding the type of care patients require and how to approach patients. But these barriers are also inherently a part of our larger healthcare system—a system that has been designed within a framework of

189

historical oppression. The system is not broken; it is working exactly as it has been designed, having been informed by heteropatriarchy, white supremacy, and capitalism. We must continue to ask complex questions about how we can completely dismantle and reimagine a system of care; that dismantling and recreation from the ashes is the goal, not the pipe dream. We must call out the exclusion of justice that is too often perpetuated on black and brown people, even when it does not advance our careers. The system as designed will continue to propagate a matrix of oppression. We ask you to consider instead that our healthcare system is doing what it has been designed to do—and therefore it must be completely dismantled, reimagined, and redesigned through a lens of racial, economic, and health justice.

At the same time, we must commit to changing the experiences that patients have with you, one on one, in the clinical setting. We as clinicians must take purposeful steps right now to build safe and trusting relationships that include activism and raising our voices to those in positions of power, in ways that should take you out of your comfort zone. This pushing against a comfort zone means that we (clinicians) are not "just here to help." We are instead here to ensure that LGBTQIA+ and BIPOC patients feel safe and entrust us with their care, knowing that we are working to create change. With such a mindset, every story they want validated, acknowledged, and seen in our clinical visits can be escalated to inform how we reimagine and redesign healthcare so the system can become inherently safe. We must not only work directly with prison healthcare providers and corrections officers to change the status quo, but we must abolish prisons. We must not only commit to spending hours on the phone with insurance companies, surgeons, and specialists to ensure essential care for those most marginalized, stigmatized, and forgotten by a system of oppression, but we must have universal healthcare.

We need to create change by:

1. Understanding the history of the pathologization that LGBTQIA+ people, particularly BIPOC people, have undergone, and the current stigma these populations experience, so that we can work to strategically address barriers
2. Creating further inclusion of LGBTQIA+ populations through provider alignment with culturally safe as well as evidence-based practices in these populations
3. Consistently accepting corrections from patients when it comes to language regarding definitions and naming of their genders, sexualities, identities, and bodies
4. Ensuring that the patient's health concerns for coming into the healthcare setting are addressed as the patient states and not the ways that create greater provider comfort
5. Utilizing this book to understand a trauma-informed approach when taking healthcare interviews and conducting physical exams in order to avoid retraumatization and allow for the greatest environment of safety by the patient
6. Recognizing the individualized and specialized needs of transgender and gender expansive (TGE) individuals during the perinatal period, including emotional and cultural needs

7. Listening and appropriately responding to your patients and their experiences
8. Choosing racial and economic justice and body autonomy as crucial points of activism, foment, and advocacy, particularly with affected communities

Despite the advice and resources this book has offered, it is important to keep in mind that this book solely offers a framework and guide. It is not a protocol for the care of patients. Much like in the context of care of different ethnic backgrounds or of any patients, for that matter, the care of LGBTQIA+ including BIPOC patients still differs from patient to patient. Understand that each patient has their own distinct narrative; a narrative that the provider must explore with the patient in order to understand how to best care for them. Receiving good healthcare is a human necessity, and if we *actually* believe that, we must put our intellects, words, compassions, deeds, intentions, careers, and selves on the line to ensure its best delivery.

Glossary

The following is a glossary of terms related to the LGBTQIA+ patient population. By familiarizing yourself with the terms, you will begin to take steps toward informed and inclusive communication. Please refer to this glossary as you read this text.

Aromantic: An individual who experiences little or no romantic attraction.

Asexual: An individual who, within the spectrum of sexuality, may not experience sexual attraction.

BDSM/Kink: *BDSM* stands for a group of erotic activities including bondage, discipline, domination, submission, sadism, and/or masochism. There are distinct subcultures under this umbrella term. *Kink* is a general term referring to being involved in sexual behavior that may be considered unique to mainstream society. Kink and BDSM are often used interchangeably to describe these behaviors, although "kink" encompasses a wider array of preferences and practices, whereas BDSM relates more to interpersonal dynamics.

Bisexual: A sexual orientation that describes a person who is emotionally, romantically, and sexually attracted to people of their own gender and people of other genders.

Cisgender: A person whose gender identity corresponds to the gender assigned at birth (in other words, a person who is not transgender).

Cisnormativity: The assumption and/or belief that all men are/should be male and all women are/should be female.

Consensual Non-Monogamy: An umbrella term used to describe relationship structures that operate outside the norms of monogamy or relationship exclusivity between two people.

Cross dresser/drag queen/drag king: These terms generally refer to those who may wear the clothing of a gender that differs from the sex they were assigned at birth for entertainment, performance, self-expression, or sexual pleasure. Some cross dressers and people who dress in drag may exhibit an overlap with components of a transgender identity. The term *transvestite* is considered pejorative.

Gay: Term used in some cultural settings to represent males who are attracted to males in a romantic, erotic, and/or emotional sense. Not all men who engage in "same sex behavior" identify as gay, and as such this label should be used with caution. This term is also used to refer to the LGBTQI (I refers to intersex) community as a whole, or as an individual identity label for anyone who does not identify as heterosexual.

Gender expansive: An adjective used to describe people who identify or express themselves in ways that broaden the culturally defined behavior or expression associated with a binary gender system.

Gender expression: The outward manner in which one individual expresses or displays their gender. This may include choices in clothing, hairstyle, speech, and/or mannerisms. Gender identity and gender expression may differ and may not conform to binary and cisgender cultural norms. Gender expression is highly personal and often changes based on need for safety and personal relationship preservation.

Gender identity: A person's internal sense of self and how they exist in the world, from the perspective of gender. This is a person's sense of being masculine, feminine, both, or neither gender. Only the person can identify this for themselves—it cannot be assigned by someone else.

Gender nonconforming: A person whose gender identity differs from that which was assigned at birth, but may be more complex, fluid, multifaceted, or otherwise less clearly defined than a transgender person. *Genderqueer* is another term used by some with this range of identities.

Gender normative: A person who by nature or by choice conforms to gender-based expectations of society.

Heteronormativity: Heteronormativity is an ideology that presumes all people have a heterosexual orientation and fit into a male/female gender binary. Heteronormativity values family traditionalism as the "normal" and correct way for people to be, and this ideology has shaped our society's norms, regulations, and laws to the present day.

Homosexual: The word *homosexual* is considered offensive as it was used as part of the American Psychiatric Association's (APA's) list of mental disorders until 1973. The Associated Press and *New York Times* style guides, for example, restrict its usage. Preferred terms are *gay, lesbian,* and *bisexual.*

Intersex: The term used for 2% of babies who are born with naturally occurring variations in chromosomes, hormones, genitalia, and other sex characteristics.

Lesbian: Term used to describe female-identified people attracted romantically, erotically, and/or emotionally to other female-identified people.

Nonbinary: Transgender or gender nonconforming person who identifies outside of the male/female gender binary; may include identities that are both male/female or neither male/female.

Pansexual: Individuals whose attractions, whether emotional or sexual, are not limited by biological sex or gender.

Polyamory: Having more than one relationship, romantic or sexual, at a time. All parties consent to the relationship structure.

Polycule: A consensually non-monogamous relationship structure.

Pronoun: A word that substitutes for a noun (e.g.: in English we can say "Jo went to the store" or we can use a pronoun and say "He or she went to the store"). Note: They/them/their are gender neutral pronouns used by some who have a nonbinary or nonconforming gender identity. If you are not in a situation to ask a patient their gender pronouns, they/them/their is preferred due to its neutrality.

Queer: The Q in LGBTQIA+. A reclaimed word that historically has been a derogatory term, but which some LGBTQIA+ people now use from a place of power and self-identity. This term is often seen as blurring the boundaries between categories of sexual orientation and gender identity and can include gay, lesbian, bisexual, and transgender identities.

Sex: The sex assigned at birth, based on assessment of external genitalia, as well as chromosomes and gonads. In everyday language it is often used interchangeably with gender; however, there are differences, which become important in the context of transgender people.

Sexual orientation: Describes sexual attraction only, and is not directly related to gender identity. The sexual orientation of transgender people should be defined by the individual. It is often described based on the lived gender; a transgender woman attracted to other women may identify as a lesbian, and a transgender man attracted to other men may identify as a gay man.

Transgender: A person whose gender identity differs from the sex that was assigned at birth. It may be abbreviated to "trans" and used as an umbrella term to describe a wide variety of gender identities including nonbinary, gender expansive, gender nonconforming, or transgender man/transgender woman. A transgender man is a person assigned female at birth who identifies as male; a transgender woman is assigned male at birth but identifies as female. A non-transgender person may be referred to as cisgender.

Trans-feminine/Transgender woman: A trans-feminine/woman has a feminine spectrum gender identity, with the sex of male assigned at birth.

Transmasculine/Transgender man: A transmasculine/man has a masculine spectrum gender identity, with the sex of female assigned at birth.

Transsexual: A more clinical term that had historically been used to describe those transgender people who sought medical intervention (i.e., hormones or surgery) for gender affirmation. This term is less commonly used in present-day; however, some individuals and communities maintain a strong and affirmative connection to this term.

RESOURCES

1. Crethar HC, Vargas LA. Multicultural intricacies in professional counseling. In: Gregoire J, Jungers C, eds. *The Counselor's Companion: What Every Beginning Counselor Needs to Know*. Lawrence Erlbaum; 2007.
2. Levine EC, Herbenick D, Martinez O, et al. Open relationships, nonconsensual nonmonogamy, and monogamy among U.S. adults: findings from the 2012 National Survey of Sexual Health and Behavior. *Arch Sex Behav*. 2018;47(5):1439–1450. doi:10.1007/s10508-018-1178-7
3. Human Rights Campaign. *Glossary of terms*. 2018. https://www.hrc.org/resources/glossary-of-terms
4. James S, Herman JL, Rankin S, et al. *The Report of the 2015 U.S. Transgender Survey*. National Center for Transgender Equality; 2015.
5. Edsall NC. *Toward Stonewall: Homosexuality and Society in the Modern Western World*. University of Virginia Press; 2003. https://muse.jhu.edu/book/16346

6. Drescher J. Queer diagnoses: parallels and contrasts in the history of homosexuality, gender variance, and the diagnostic and statistical manual. *Arch Sex Behav*. 2010;39(2):427–460. doi:10.1007/s10508-009-9531-5

7. Sheff E, Wolf T. *Stories From the Polycule: Real Life in Polyamorous Families*. Thorntree Press; 2015.

8. Grant MM. Learning, beliefs, and products: students' perspectives with project-based learning. *Interdiscip J Probl Based Learn*. 2011;5(2). doi:10.7771/1541-5015.1254

9. Baker K, Beagan B. Making assumptions, making space: an anthropological critique of cultural competency and its relevance to queer patients: making assumptions, making space. *Med Anthropol Q*. 2014;28(4):578–598. doi:10.1111/maq.12129

10. Goins ES, Pye D. Check the box that best describes you: reflexively managing theory and praxis in LGBTQ health communication research. *Health Commun*. 2013;28(4):397–407. doi:10.1080/10410236.2012.690505

11. Phelan SM, Burgess DJ, Yeazel MW, et al. Impact of weight bias and stigma on quality of care and outcomes for patients with obesity. *Obes Rev*. 2015;16(4):319–326. doi:10.1111/obr.12266

12. Hall EV, Galinsky AD, Phillips KW. Gender profiling: a gendered race perspective on person–position fit. *Pers Soc Psychol Bull*. 2015;41(6):853–868. doi:10.1177/0146167215580779

13. van Ryn M, Hardeman R, Phelan SM, et al. Medical school experiences associated with change in implicit racial bias among 3547 students: a medical student CHANGES study report. *J Gen Intern Med*. 2015;30(12):1748–1756. doi:10.1007/s11606-015-3447-7

14. Makadon HJ, Mayer KH, Potter J, et al., eds. *The Fenway Guide to Lesbian, Gay, Bisexual, and Transgender Health*. 2nd ed. American College of Physicians; 2015.

15. Dubin SN, Nolan IT, Streed CG Jr, et al. Transgender health care: improving medical students' and residents' training and awareness. *Adv Med Educ Pract*. 2018;9:377–391. doi:10.2147/AMEP.S147183

16. Human Rights Campaign. Sexual orientation and gender identity definitions. 2015. http://www.hrc.org/resources/entry/sexual-orientation-and-gender-identity-terminology-and-definitions

17. Singer R. LGBTQ training for obstetrical care providers in two urban settings: an examination of changes in knowledge, attitude and intended behavior. Published March 2016. https://search.proquest.com/openview/9951081849d694ffbbb8965e261dbe13/1?pq-origsite=gscholar&cbl=18750&diss=y

18. Mountz S, Capous-Desyllas M, Pourciau E. "Because we're fighting to be ourselves": voices from former foster youth who are transgender and gender expansive. *Child Welf*. 2018;96(1):103. https://www.researchgate.net/publication/326464141_'Because_We're_Fighting_to_Be_Ourselves'_Voices_from_Former_Foster_Youth_who_are_Transgender_and_Gender_Expansive

19. Gamarel KE, Brown L, Kahler CW, et al. Prevalence and correlates of substance use among youth living with HIV in clinical settings. *Drug Alcohol Depend*. 2016;169:11–18. doi:10.1016/j.drugalcdep.2016.10.002

20. Pan, L, Moore A. Gender unicorn. http://www.transstudent.org/gender

21. Intersex Society of North America. http://www.isna.org

22. Richards C, Barker MJ. *The Palgrave Handbook of the Psychology of Sexuality and Gender*. Palgrave Macmillan; 2015.

23. Oswald RF, Blume LB, Marks S. Decentering heteronormativity: a model for family studies. In: Bengtson VL, Acock AC, Allen KR, eds. *Sourcebook of Family Theory and Research*. SAGE Publications Inc.; 2005.

Index

Printed in the United States
by Hignell Book Printing Services

Printed in the United States
by Baker & Taylor Publisher Services